Y0-ABZ-342

Robt T Beck

THE EXPLORATION OF THE INNER WORLD

THE EXPLORATION OF THE INNER WORLD

A Study of Mental Disorder and Religious Experience

BY

ANTON T. BOISEN

*Research Associate in the Psychology of Religion
and Chaplain, the Elgin (Ill.) State Hospital;
Lecturer, the Chicago Theological Seminary*

WILLETT, CLARK & COMPANY
CHICAGO   NEW YORK
1936

TO THE MEMORY

OF

A. L. B.

For her sake I undertook the adventure out of which this book has grown. Her compassion upon a wretch in direst need, her wisdom and courage and unswerving fidelity have made possible the measure of success which may have been achieved. To her I dedicate it in the name of the Love which would surmount every barrier, and bridge every chasm and make sure the foundations of the universe.

CONTENTS

FOR THE GUIDANCE OF THE READER

THE DISTINCTIVE feature of this book lies in its attempt to study the experiences of inner defeat and of inner victory, the one in the light of the other. It makes the hypothesis that there is an important relationship between acute mental illness of the functional type and those sudden transformations of character so prominent in the history of the Christian church since the days of Saul of Tarsus. It undertakes to show that both may arise out of a common situation — that of inner conflict and disharmony, accompanied by a keen awareness of ultimate loyalties and unattained possibilities. Religious experience as well as mental disorder may involve severe emotional upheaval, and mental disorder as well as religious experience may represent the operation of the healing forces of nature. The conclusion follows that certain types of mental disorder and certain types of religious experience are alike attempts at reorganization. The difference lies in the outcome. Where the attempt is successful and some degree of victory is won, it is commonly recognized as religious experience. Where it is unsuccessful or indeterminate, it is commonly spoken of as "insanity." In those constructive transformations of the personality which we recognize as religious experience, the individual is relieved of his sense of isolation and is brought into harmony with that which is supreme in his hierarchy of loyalties. He succeeds in effecting a synthesis between the crisis experience and his subsequent life which enables him to grow in the direction of inner unification and social adaptation on a basis conceived as universal. In most of those cases which we speak of as "mental illness," no such synthesis is achieved. The patient may get well but he may not solve his problem. Frequently he becomes stabilized on an unsatisfactory basis, or else he becomes increasingly discouraged and disorganized.

A further feature of this book lies in the fact that I approach the problem not merely as a specialist in both the psychology and sociology of religion but also in psychopathology. What is more, I come to it as one who has personally explored the little-known country with which it deals. It was by passing, myself, through a brief but extremely severe period of mental illness that my attention was drawn to the problem. This occurred in my forty-fourth year. Previous to that time I had, during my seminary course, done special work in the psychology of religion under the direction of Professor George A. Coe. I had put several years into the making of social and religious surveys and I had served as a rural pastor. Following the period of mental illness I spent two and a half years in graduate study at Harvard University under Dr. Macfie Campbell, Dr. Richard C. Cabot and Professor William McDougall. I then went to the Worcester State Hospital in Massachusetts. I believe that I can claim that my eight years' service as chaplain of that institution was the first attempt to bring to such a position any special training for the service of the mentally ill. I have now since 1932 been serving as chaplain at the Elgin State Hospital in Illinois. Since 1925 I have been on the faculty of the Chicago Theological Seminary as research associate and lecturer in psychopathology. Results of studies which I have made in this field have appeared in various scientific journals. The substance of what is contained in the chapter on "The Wilderness of the Lost" appeared in the *American Journal of Psychiatry* for November, 1933. The chapter on "The Battleground of Character" embodies the substance of two articles, one of which appeared in the *American Journal of Psychiatry* for 1926 and the other in the *American Journal of Sociology* for 1928. The chapter on "The Problem of Right and Wrong" is adapted from an article in the *American Journal of Sociology* for 1932. In addition to this research work I have initiated a plan for the clinical training of theological students which is now organized on a national basis and has given training to some three hundred students.

In writing this book I have been embarrassed by the fact that the field which it covers is divided into two distinct sections, each of which is presided over by a professional group which has its own vocabulary, and neither of which knows much about the other. The nature of my problem and the purpose of my book require that I write with both these groups in mind. The difficulty is increased by the fact that as a traveler reporting on a little-known country, it is incumbent upon me to give an accurate account of the territory which I have explored. So far as possible I have sought to use simple and nontechnical language, but there are sections in which the reader may have to shift gears. Thus in the chapter on "The Wilderness of the Lost," which represents ten years of research work and provides the foundation of all that follows, the requirements of accuracy and closeness of reasoning have seemed to me paramount. I trust however that the problem dealt with will be of sufficient importance that the reader will bear with a little unfamiliar phraseology, and that the book will be of interest not merely to psychiatrists and students of religion, but also to students of the psychological and social sciences and to intelligent laymen who may be grappling with the problems of which it treats. To meet the difficulty I have provided in the Appendix a list of the more important technical terms and concepts which will serve not merely as a glossary but as a review of the two major fields under consideration.

While I have sought to make the book as concrete and interesting as I knew how, it will be clear that my purpose has not been to produce a popular book. We have already enough of these in this field. My reason for writing it is to offer a new contribution to an important human problem. In Part I, I present a survey of the fields of mental illness and of religious experience and draw from this certain generalizations. Part II deals with the theoretical implications. These include the problem of religious genius as represented supremely in Jesus of Nazareth, the determinants of character, the problem of right and wrong and the laws with which theology has to do. Part III is an attempt to apply the principles thus arrived at to the work of the churches and of the minister of religion. In thus limiting the application to the one professional group and their constituency, I am guided by considerations of modesty. It has not seemed to me fitting that I should offer suggestions to any professional group other than the one to which I belong.

For my thesis I think I can claim that it is independent and distinctive. Certainly I have ample reason to know that the relationship which I am pointing out between the domain of mental illness and that of religious experience has thus far been strangely ignored by both psychiatrists and theologians. If that relationship can be established there should be far-reaching consequences.

It is a pleasure to acknowledge my indebtedness to my colleagues, Professor Arthur E. Holt, Professor Fred Eastman and Professor A. C. Mc-Giffert, with whom I have consulted throughout the preparation of the manuscript. Others who have read the manuscript and have offered valuable suggestions are Dr. Helen Flanders Dunbar, Dr. Charles F. Read, Reverend Donald C. Beatty, Professor George A. Coe, Dr. Macfie Campbell, Dr. R. G. Hoskins and Professor A. R. Radcliffe-Brown. Professor Henry J. Cadbury and Dr. Harry Stack Sullivan have helped me with certain portions of the manuscript. To the editors and publishers of the *American Journal of Psychiatry* and of the *American Journal of Sociology* I am indebted for permission to use material which appeared originally in their pages.

A. T. B.

Elgin, Illinois
August, 1936

THE EXPLORATION OF THE INNER WORLD

INTRODUCTION

To be plunged as a patient into a hospital for the insane may be a tragedy or it may be an opportunity. For me it has been an opportunity. It has introduced to me a new world of absorbing interest and profound significance; it has shown me that world throughout its entire range, from the bottommost depths of the nether regions to the heights of religious experience at its best; it has made me aware of certain relationships between two important fields of human experience which thus far have been held strictly apart; and it has given me a task in which I find the meaning and purpose of my life.

Sixteen years ago such possibilities were entirely undreamed of. Thus in the year 1920 I was riding on a train in the state of North Dakota when I noticed off to the south a large group of buildings standing in sharp relief against the horizon. I inquired of my neighbor in the seat what those buildings were. He informed me that I was looking at the State Insane Asylum. I thanked him and thought no more about it. It did not occur to me that I ought to be interested in those buildings or in the problem which they represented. And yet there were certain reasons why I ought to have been interested. During my course at the Union Theological Seminary nine years before I had centered my attention upon the study of the psychology of religion with particular reference to the problem of mysticism. And at that very time I was in charge of a sociological survey of the state under the direction of the Interchurch World Movement, and as a part of my task I was investigating the situation as regards church hospitals. Probably I should have remained uninterested for some time longer, if, less than a year later, I had not found myself plunged as a patient within the confines of just such an institution.

While it is not my purpose to tell how this happened, I shall give a few facts which will make clear the point of view from which this inquiry has been approached and also the biases which will influence my findings. The disturbance came on very suddenly and it was extremely severe. I had never been in better condition physically; the difficulty was rooted wholly in a severe inner struggle arising out of a precocious sexual sensitivity, dating from my fourth year. With the onset of adolescence the struggle became quite severe. It was cleared up on Easter morning in my twenty-second year through a spontaneous religious conversion experience which followed upon a period of black despair. An impulse, seemingly from without myself, bade me not to be afraid to tell. I was thus set free and given a new start in life. Two years later came a relapse into the land of bondage and then a desperate struggle to get free again. Following a decision to give up the teaching of languages, in which I was then engaged, and to enter upon the profession of forestry, there came a love affair which swept me off my feet and sent me forth on the adventure which has resulted in this book. This love affair was on my part a desperate cry for salvation. It led to my decision to enter the Christian ministry. The woman I loved was a religious worker of the finest type. On her part it was a source of great embarrassment, but she gave me a helping hand at the critical moment and stood ready to undertake what for her was a task of mercy. But I failed to make the grade. Then followed nine years of wandering. This included several years in rural survey work, five years in the rural pastorate and two with the Y.M.C.A. overseas. On my return I had charge of a state survey for the Interchurch World Movement. All this time I was hoping to be reinstated with her. It was as though my life depended upon it. In 1920 such a reinstatement did occur. The disturbance followed shortly after, coming thus just at the time when the hopes of so many years seemed about to be realized.

I had had, when the Interchurch World Movement disbanded,

an enticing opportunity to go on with the survey work. This I had turned down, having decided definitely to go back into the pastorate. I wanted to work out what I felt to be my religious message. The call to a church was slow in coming and I went east. While waiting I decided to write out a statement of my religious experience, such as I had been required to do when I was a candidate for ordination. I became much absorbed in the task, so much so that I lay awake at night letting the ideas take shape of themselves, as I frequently do when I am writing. This time the ideas carried me away. First of all came the thought that I must give up the hope which meant everything to me. Following this there came surging in upon me with overpowering force a terrifying idea about a coming world catastrophe. Although I had never before given serious thought to such a subject, there came flashing into my mind, as though from a source without myself, the idea that this little planet of ours, which has existed for we know not how many millions of years, was about to undergo some sort of metamorphosis. It was like a seed or an egg. In it were stored up a quantity of food materials, represented by our natural resources. But now we were like a seed in the process of germinating or an egg that had just been fertilized. We were starting to grow. Just within the short space of a hundred years we had begun to draw upon our resources to such an extent that the timber and the gas and the oil were likely soon to be exhausted. In the wake of this idea followed others. I myself was more important than I had ever dreamed of being; I was also a zero quantity. Strange and mysterious forces of evil of which before I had not had the slightest suspicion were also revealed. I was terrified beyond measure and in my terror I talked. Of course my family was frightened and I soon found myself in a psychopathic hospital. There followed three weeks of violent delirium which remain indelibly burned into my memory. There is probably no three-weeks period in all my life that I can recall more clearly. It seemed as if I were living thousands of years within that time. Then I came out of it much as one awakens out of a bad dream.

I remember distinctly one incident which helped me to find my way out. The idea which had first bowled me over was, as I have said, that of a coming world catastrophe. This same idea was dominant throughout as the premise on which my reasoning was based. I was therefore much impressed one night, as I lay awake out on the sleeping-porch, by the observation that the moon was centered in a cross of light. I took this as confirmation of my worst fears. Did not the cross stand for suffering? What else could it mean than this, that the moon — which, as so often happens in acute disturbances, I had personified — is in mourning over the coming doom? In order to be sure I called an attendant and inquired if he also saw the cross. He said that he did. I was greatly impressed and agitated. But some days later in the early watches of the morning as I lay awake looking at the moon, speculating about the terrible danger which that cross betokened, I made a discovery. Whenever I looked at the moon from a certain spot the cross did not appear. I immediately investigated and found that from that particular spot I was looking at the moon through a hole in the wire screening! With this discovery the edifice I had reared upon the basis of the original premise began to fall. And only a few days later I was well again.

Concerning the severity of the disturbance I may say that the diagnosis was " catatonic dementia praecox " and that my people were told there was no hope of recovery. In consequence, when I did recover I had difficulty in convincing them that I was well enough to leave, and my stay in the hospital was for this reason longer than it would otherwise have been. I may also say that during those three weeks I lost thirty pounds in weight, but three weeks after I had made the discovery in regard to the moon I had nearly gained it back and felt physically as fit as ever. And I was also fit mentally except for certain lurking fears which I stowed away in the back of my mind with a question mark after them.

Very naturally I became interested during the days that followed in the attempt to find out just what had happened to me. I began by observing my fellow patients. I soon learned that there was a group of them that once each week took certain treatments. It seemed that they had a disease called " general paresis."

There was one young man who had something the nurse called "post-encephalitis." She explained that this also had an organic basis. Then there were several old men on the ward, some of whom had hardening of the arteries in the brain. But aside from these my fellow patients seemed well enough physically. And some I met who had been inmates of the hospital for twenty-five, thirty, and even forty years, all the time apparently in good physical health. But they were on the whole a rather discouraged lot of men. I arrived at the conclusion that what had happened to me had happened also to them. Their inner world had come crashing down. They had perhaps been thinking intently on something until they had put themselves into an abnormal condition. I came also to the conclusion that the particular thing most of them had been concerned about was of the same general nature as that which caused some people to "hit the sawdust trail" at the meetings of evangelists like Billy Sunday. It came over me like a flash that if inner conflicts like that which Paul describes in the famous passage in the seventh chapter of Romans can have happy solutions, as the church has always believed, there must also be unhappy solutions which thus far the church has ignored. It came to me that what I was being faced with in the hospital were the unhappy solutions. Most of the patients whom I saw around me would then be in the hospital because of spiritual or religious difficulties.

Of course I spent much time puzzling about my own case. I tried to get a chance to talk with the doctor about it. In this I met with little success. That particular hospital took the organicist point of view. The doctors did not believe in talking with patients about their symptoms, which they assumed to be rooted in some as yet undiscovered organic difficulty. The longest time I ever got was fifteen minutes during which the very charming young doctor pointed out that one must not hold the reins too tight in dealing with the sex instinct. Nature, he said, must have its way. It was very clear that he had neither understanding nor interest in the religious aspects of my problem.

I was very happy to find that there were religious services on

Sunday afternoons. But I soon discovered that the ministers from the neighboring village who conducted those services might know something about religion, but they certainly knew nothing about our problems. They did no visiting on the wards — which may not have been entirely their fault, as they probably received little encouragement to do so. All they did was to conduct a formal service on Sunday afternoons, and for lack of anything better they usually gave us the same sermons they had given their own congregations in the morning. There was one kindly old minister who gave us a series of sermons on missions — missions in China, missions in Africa, missions in Japan. Another preached on the text, " If thine eye offend thee, pluck it out." I was afraid that one or two of my fellow patients might be inclined to take that injunction literally.

For four and a half months I gave most of my attention to the attempt to understand my experience and also to convince my friends that I was as well as I had ever been. But the harder I tried the less they believed it. The result was to increase my own fears and my own sense of helplessness. There followed then another period of disturbance quite as severe as the first and ten weeks in duration instead of three. This also began suddenly and ended abruptly. On coming out of it, I changed my tactics and said nothing about release. Instead I looked around for something to do. I was struck by the number of patients in my ward who spent most of the day sitting still, looking off into the distance and thinking apparently very gloomy thoughts. I suggested some games in which it might be possible to interest them. I ventured to suggest and write out a program for a play festival on the " Glorious Fourth " which was then about three weeks in the offing. I also looked around for a regular job and suggested several things I should enjoy doing, among them wood-working and photography. It so happened that they wanted someone to do photographic work, so they gave me the job. It will be seen that the doctors were really kind and responsive and that I did find something to do that I could enjoy. And I had an opportunity to study the hospital inside and out.

The question of what to do with myself after I left the hospital was of course a knotty problem. I myself had a very definite idea of what I wanted to do. I had not been three weeks out of the psychopathic ward before I was clear on that. The new-formed purpose was expressed as follows in a letter of February 14, 1921:

This catastrophe has of course destroyed my hopes and my plans. I came back east in July with the intention of taking a pastorate. From that, I take it, I am now turned aside. My present purpose is to take as my problem the one with which I am now confronted, the service of these unfortunates with whom I am surrounded. I feel that many forms of insanity are religious rather than medical problems and that they cannot be successfully treated until they are so recognized. The problem seems to me one of great importance not only because of the large number who are now suffering from mental ailments but also because of its religious and psychological and philosophical aspects. I am very sure that if I can make to it any contribution whatsoever it will be worth the cost.

There were of course many difficulties to be overcome. The doctors did not favor it. My friends had to be convinced, and that was no easy task. Some even thought it was my duty to remain in the hospital as a patient for the rest of my life. Others assumed that something in the nature of simple manual work was all that would now be open to me. The following letter, written on August 14, 1921, will give an idea of the situation with which I was confronted at that time:

I am quite cheered by the fact that my cherished plan for the coming year meets with your approval. . . .

I had a most welcome visit the other day from my old friend P. who has now an important church in M——. P. brought with him some good advice which he hatched out coming down on the train. He thought that some work which would keep me right down to concrete things would be the best way to regain or retain my sanity! I said to him: " Hang the sanity! You can't ever make life worth living if all you're doing is to try to keep from going insane. The object of life is to accomplish things worth while, to solve problems and to make contributions of some sort to this world in which we live. As I see it, a man ought to be willing to go through Hell if thereby he has even a chance of doing something which is really worth doing."

This reminds me of a little incident from my forestry days. One day during my sojourn in Washington in 1907, I walked into one of the rooms in the Forest Service Building and found there quite a little gathering. One of our old classmates at Yale had just returned from two years up in the north woods and was busily engaged in dishing out yarns about his experience in the wilds. One of the questions and its answer I'll never forget. " Say, Bill," asked one of the group, " have you ever been lost? " Bill straightened up, glared at him and replied with some heat: " Lost? Of course I've been. It's only the dubs who never go five miles from camp, who don't get lost sometimes." Now I do not mean to imply that those who do keep their poise and their sanity are able to do so only because they never venture off the beaten path. I only mean that for me to stick right to camp and wash dishes all the rest of my life for fear of getting lost again would take out of life all that makes it worth living for me. I am not afraid. I have always managed to find my way through; and I do think that in a very real sense I have been exploring some little-known territory which I should like now to have a chance to map out.

In the end my plan went through. My mother gave her consent, conditioned upon the approval of Dr. Elwood Worcester. With him I had a series of helpful conferences which have left me with a high opinion of his insight and wisdom. In February, 1922, I enrolled for special work in the Andover Theological Seminary and in the graduate school of Harvard University. I was fortunate enough to be included in Dr. Macfie Campbell's seminar at the Boston Psychopathic Hospital. I found much help also in some work I took with Dr. Richard C. Cabot. The following year I continued my work with these men together also with Professor William McDougall. At the end of the second year I looked around for an opening. I wanted a chaplaincy in a hospital. I soon discovered that there were no such jobs. What is more, the hospital superintendents were not enthusiastic over the idea. I even tried to get a job as attendant with the stipulation that I might have access to the case records. But that stipulation barred me out.

The year 1923-24 was therefore spent at the Boston Psychopathic Hospital. I worked during the summer in the psychological department under Dr. F. L. Wells. In the fall I transferred to the social service department under Miss Susie Lyons. Here I found just the opportunity I was looking for to study cases from all angles. From the standpoint of one who had spent three years in the making of sociological surveys, I made an interesting discovery. Before, as a mere inquirer, I had had to stop at the very points in which as a student of religion I was most interested. I did not dare in my survey work to inquire into the moral conditions or the inner experiences of the people. I would not have got anywhere if I had. But now I was beginning with precisely those problems embodied in the cases of individuals in difficulty. And because my purpose was that of helping those individuals rather than that of mere inquiry the friends were ready to talk, and I received insights into the social situation otherwise impossible. In the course of this work at the Psychopathic Hospital I became interested in certain of the missions in the Negro section in Roxbury and most of the last four months was spent in making a special study of their activities and influence.

The next year there came an opening at the Worcester State Hospital. In Dr. William A. Bryan I found a superintendent who rejoices in making it possible for men with very different points of view to work together at the same problem. He did indeed have to put up with a good bit of chaffing from his fellow superintendents for such an unheard-of innovation as that of bringing a full-time chaplain into a mental hospital. This he met with the reply that he would be perfectly willing to bring in a horse doctor if he thought there was any chance of his being able to help the patients.

In the spring of 1925 through my friend, Professor Arthur E. Holt, who has done more than anyone else to help me in getting the new start, there came an opening as research associate in the Chicago Theological Seminary. I spent the fall quarter there. My first task was an experiment in a small mining community near La Salle. I sought to approach from my point of view the problems of some ordinary group of people such as the minister has to deal with. The time was too short to accomplish much in the way of results beyond the new insights into pastoral work and its possibilities which it gave me. The following fall quarter I had my first course at the seminary and until the fall of 1930 I continued to spend three months of each year in Chicago.

In the summer of 1925 I was given the opportunity to try the experiment of bringing some theological students to the hospital. These students worked on the wards as ordinary attendants. My own experience had convinced me that there is no one upon whom the patient's welfare is more dependent than the nurse or attendant who is with him hour after hour during the day. I felt also that such work provided an unequaled opportunity to observe and understand the patient, and I was much concerned that theological students should have the opportunity to go to first-hand sources for their knowledge of human nature. I wanted them to learn to read human documents as well as books, particularly those revealing documents which are opened up at the inner day of judgment. These students were allowed to have information in regard to the cases. They were permitted to attend the medical staff meetings and for their benefit we held special conferences. There were four students the first summer. The plan was sufficiently successful to warrant another trial. Since then the number has increased rapidly and whatever success my undertaking has had at Worcester and at Elgin as well has been due to the fine work of these students and the favorable impression they have left upon the hospital community.

During the last week in November, 1920, three weeks after I had made my little discovery in regard to the moon, I had written a long letter setting forth my explanation of what had happened to me. I had at this time done no reading whatever in psychiatric literature and I did not even know that such a man as Freud existed. The conclusions were drawn entirely from my own experience and observations in the light of the work I had previously done in the psychology of religion. In the years that have followed the original hypothesis has been considerably modified and elaborated, but in its essence it remains unchanged as the working hypothesis which has determined all my subsequent work. The following paragraph from that letter may be taken as the thesis of this book:

As I look around me here and then try to analyze my own case, I see two main classes of insanity. In the one case there is some organic trouble, a defect in the brain tissue, some disorder in the nervous system, some disease of the blood. In the other there is no organic difficulty. The body is strong and the brain in good working order. The difficulty is rather in the *disorganization of the patient's world*. Something has happened which has upset the foundations upon which his ordinary reasoning is based. Death or disappointment or sense of failure may have compelled a reconstruction of the patient's world view from the bottom up, and the mind becomes dominated by the one idea which he has been trying to put in its proper place. That, I think, has been my trouble and I think it is the trouble with many others also.

In the pages that follow I propose to examine, in the light of my own experience, the experience of other persons who have been forced off the beaten path of common sense and have traveled through the little-known wilderness of the inner life. I shall seek, so far as possible, to arrive at some comprehensive view of this inner world throughout its entire range. I shall examine not only the unhappy solutions of inner conflicts but also the happy ones. This I shall do with the ever deepening conviction that only as we study the one in the light of the other shall we be able to understand either one or to gain any insight into the laws of the spiritual life with which theology and psychiatry are equally concerned.

Any value that this study may have will lie primarily in the fact that it is a report of one who has himself explored the country which he describes, one who has passed through an experience which was at once mental disorder of the most profound and unmistakable variety and also, for himself at least, of unquestionable religious value. For the same reason this study will be subject to the inevitable biases of the participant observer.

While I do not consider it wise to enter into the more personal factors in my own case, I shall feel myself free to make use of observations and conclusions made at the time of my initiation into this realm of the lower regions, believing that these may have some value in that they were arrived at independently on the basis of my own personal experience and observations with relatively little influence by the views and theories of other men.

PART I

A JOURNEY OF EXPLORATION

I

THE WILDERNESS OF THE LOST

SHORTLY AFTER my arrival at Worcester I was waited upon by a committee of young men from the Worcester Institute of Technology. They came to invite me to speak to their student forum. Their invitation I was happy to accept. Then came the question, What will the subject be? " You know," explained the leader of the delegation, " we must have a title with punch in it if we are to expect the fellows to come." Here was a problem for which I was unprepared, so he came to my rescue. " Why not call it," he suggested, " The Place Where You Are Going by One Who Is There "? We finally agreed that this title might not be altogether flattering to my audience and that " A Message from Purgatory " would suit somewhat better. I have used that title a number of times since then with an increasing belief in its essential accuracy. Certainly it is the lower regions with which we are to begin our exploration of the inner world.

Over the gates of his Inferno Dante Alighieri saw the legend, " All hope abandon, ye who enter here." As I read the *Divine Comedy* and the *Vita Nuova,* I get the impression that Dante himself had explored very thoroughly this inner world and that he has given us a marvelous first-hand account of what he saw. But he was perhaps too much influenced by medieval theology. At least I find no evidence of any hell of eternal torment, and the pictures which he gives us of what he saw within that ominous gate contain too much of suffering and agony to accord with that inscription. Suffering, as I see it, is remedial. As long as there is suffering there is hope. When hope departs pain and suffering also leave. I shall therefore consider together both purgatory and the region from which there is no return. For this procedure there is a further reason in that I find them both combined in those experiences which are grouped together under the same general label which was affixed to my own case.

For such a study I have had an unusual opportunity. In the spring of 1927 there began at Worcester an exhaustive study of this precise group of cases. This study was conducted primarily from the standpoint of the endocrinologist under the direct supervision of one of the foremost specialists in the country, Dr. Roy G. Hoskins of the Harvard Medical School, director of the Memorial Foundation for Neuro-Endocrine Research and editor-in-chief of the *Journal of Endocrinology*. I have had the good fortune to be associated with this project from the time it began and I have received much help and encouragement from Dr. Hoskins and his associates. While concerned primarily with the physiological factors they have sought to approach the problem from all possible angles and have recognized that whatever the organic basis of dementia praecox may be it is to the sufferer himself primarily an experience. They have therefore given me a free hand in my approach to the problem and it has been no small privilege to be able to use for the basis of this study cases which have been exhaustively studied from the physiological angle. The close observations which have been made on behavior and ideation in these cases by the members of the research staff have also been of greatest value. So far as possible the 173 cases used in this study have been taken serially from the research group, thus avoiding the danger of a selective bias on my part. The only exceptions were a few cases in which my data were inadequate.

To the knowledge of the behavior and ideation of these patients I have been able to make some contribution through the results obtained by the use of a ward observation blank worked out originally for the use of my students in their work as attendants on the wards. Over a period of three years this was used by special

observers, all of whom were selected from among my students. I
have also interviewed most of the patients with the aid of a list of
questions based upon the analysis of the thought content found
in the first eighty cases.[1] These questions have proved most helpful in gaining access to the mind of the patient and revealing his
significant ideas. In some cases I have done intensive therapeutic
work and have made social investigations.

In accordance with the plan adopted by those in charge of the
research project, the great majority of the patients chosen for study
have been males of less than forty years of age whose cases have
been uncomplicated by gross organic disease. Many of these
patients had been in the hospital for a considerable period of time.
Of the 173 used in this study 22 had in 1931 been in the hospital
less than one year, 23 from one to two years, 26 from two to three
years, 44 from three to five years, 40 from six to ten years, and
18 for more than ten years.[2] More than one-third of the cases
chosen for study and experimental therapy have thus been in the
hospital for six years or longer and the series is heavily weighted
with cases of the chronic type. In consequence the odds are very
great against a high recovery rate. A series of newly admitted
patients would give very different results.

This group of patients have been given intensive study and treatment. They have been placed on special wards with a full and

---

[1] For this list of questions I am indebted to Dr. Helen F. Dunbar.

[2] An examination of the records yields the following additional data which may help
to give an idea of the type represented:

The age groupings show 9 patients under 21 years of age, 75 between 21 and 30 years,
61 between 31 and 40 years, and 28 of more than 40 years.

In the matter of schooling 37 have had sixth grade education or less, 65 have been
through seventh or eighth grade; 27 have stopped with first or second year high school
and 26 have gone as far as third or fourth year high school; 18 have had more or less
college training.

Racially we find 39 Irish, 34 English, 20 French Canadian, 11 Hebrew, 7 Slavic, 6
German, 3 Negro, and a scattering among a dozen or more other races. Ecclesiastically
101 are Roman Catholics, 57 are Protestants, 11 Hebrew, 4 Greek Orthodox, and 1
Mohammedan.

Under marital conditions we find 142 single, 24 married, 4 divorced, 2 widowed,
and 1 unknown.

Occupationally 46 are listed as common laborers, 19 as mill-hands, 14 machinists,
15 bookkeepers or clerks, 14 students, 6 farm-hands, and 3 professional men. Ten have
never had any occupation. The rest are scattering.

carefully selected staff of nurses and attendants. They have been given carefully controlled glandular medication over a long period of time. They have received special medical and psychiatric attention and special provision has been made for recreational and occupational therapy. Everything possible has been done to strengthen the morale and to deal constructively with personal problems. Not only have conferences been held at frequent intervals with individual patients, but there have been group conferences for selected patients. One of the most interesting experiments is that of posting at regular intervals the ratings of the patients according to a system of classification which has been carefully worked out and explained to them.[3] The effort has been made constantly to stimulate pride, to foster self-respect, to provide incentives and to give recognition to each forward step. And these efforts have in some instances been continued for more than four years.

This group of cases is not sufficiently large to give well rounded graphs, but it may suffice to show that my own experience is by no means an isolated one. It may also provide a basis for checking and elaborating my hypothesis that such experiences are to be explained in terms of the disorganization of the inner world consequent upon the upsetting of the foundations upon which the critical judgments are made and that, as such, it is closely related to certain types of religious experience.

Our first task will involve the use of statistics. It requires the checking of the hypothesis derived first of all from my own experience and then from intensive work with certain other cases against this group of 173 cases. This I propose to do in the light of a particular experience which may be used as a sort of base line from which our measurements may be taken. In this way there will be less danger that we lose sight of human values. We shall also be less likely to become confused as to what we are talking about, for concrete experience can to a large extent serve as substitute for an exactness of definition not yet warranted by the

[3] Cf. R. G. Hoskins and M. H. Erickson, " The Grading of Patients in Mental Hospitals as a Therapeutic Measure." *American Journal of Psychiatry,* II, 103–9.

adequacy of knowledge. The following case has been chosen as suited to our purpose:

Albert W., a migrant laborer of thirty years, with seventh grade education and fair intelligence, who was brought to our hospital in an acutely disturbed condition, had had about all the handicaps that a boy can have in the matter of heredity and early influences. Both his parents and also his paternal grandfather had been alcoholic. The parents had in fact carried their alcoholic proclivities to such lengths as to be committed to state institutions, and Albert from his fourth year on had been a state ward. In this rôle he had been very troublesome. He was persistently dishonest, disobedient, untruthful and quarrelsome. He was likewise a poor student. After being shunted around from one foster home to another, all the time unhappy and friendless, he was committed as a delinquent child to a reform school. Here he remained two years. After leaving the reform school, he drifted from one job to another and finally became a migrant laborer. As such he wandered over the country doing a great variety of work and at times making good wages. He thus worked seven months as an electrician in Ford's factory in Detroit and four months in the Cadillac factory. His best pay was earned as a strikebreaker. His earnings he spent freely. Gambling and women accounted for a good portion of them. And much of the time he was out of work.

According to his own story he had begun autoerotic practices at the age of fourteen and had worried a good deal about it. At fifteen he had had his first heterosexual experience. At the reform school he had run into homosexual practices which the boys called " pumpkin-scraping." He admits definite homosexual tendencies. He speaks of his morals as having reached the " x y level ", and of " associating with women whose morals were no better." Three or four years before his admission he had a serious love affair with the sister of his brother-in-law. The termination of this affair left him deeply depressed.

Heredity and environment could hardly have been much worse, and yet we find in this boy a certain fine social sensitivity. At the staff meeting he spoke of himself as having always had an " aposto-galia." Asked what that meant, he explained that it was a word which he had coined himself from the Greek to mean " following an ideal." It was brought out at this staff meeting that for six years preceding admission he had been devoting himself to solid reading and serious thinking worthy of a college-bred philosopher. This idealistic tendency had shown itself in his unhappy boy-hood in his idealization of his worthless parents. It had received its special impetus in the influence of the radicals and I.W.W.'s on the road. Stimulated by their discussions he had begun to frequent the libraries. According to his own story, whenever he came to a new town the first thing he looked for was a lodging place and the second a library. He states that he had spent on the average some two or three hours a day in those libraries, reading, not fiction, but philosophy and psychology and theology and sociology and poetry. Much of that reading he seemed really to have assimilated.

Two months before his admission he began to feel that some-thing strange was going on and he went to the police to straighten things out. He told them of his court record and asked them to investigate charges which were being made against him. They obligingly took him into custody but finding no basis for his sus-picions they dismissed him. He continued his wanderings, be-coming more and more disturbed until he felt himself " in posses-sion of a power that he didn't have before." He then began to have " a flood of mental pictures as though an album were un-folding itself." He next became terror-stricken. He had a vision of a dark woman who seemed to be supernatural. She came and hovered over him and announced that it was time for him to follow her. He became overwhelmed with fear of the unknown. He thought he was going to die. Then he saw things in a new light. The trees took on a different appearance and it came to him that " the dawn of creation " had come. Communications came to him " from out of the ether " which impressed him with the feeling that there was a great " I and You contest " going on. It came to him that he had lived before this present life. At one time he had been Jonah. He had also been St. Augustine. And he had been Christ. During his severe disturbance he thought of himself at times as roaming around the universe. But he was particularly concerned with this solar system. The sun meant to him paradise. It was associated with the idea of God. The moon was inhabited and the moon men were " in cahoots " with the men of this world. Each individual in the world had a prototype in the moon and if anyone on earth was in a hard fix, he was welcomed to the moon but a moon man must take his place here.

At the hospital, after the emotional disturbance passed, he made a good adjustment. He was given a ground parole and showed himself co-operative and dependable. He had a delightful sense of humor and a gift for expressing himself in clear and picturesque language. The disturbance was to him at this time a religious experience, something which had given him new life and hope.

The final outcome was not however a happy one. Shortly after discovering him and beginning to see him regularly I had to be absent for three months. On my return he was found disturbed and antagonistic. He had run away from the hospital to New York City. There he had suffered another upset from which he has not emerged but has remained suspicious and gloomy and inaccessible.

This case is representative of the acutely disturbed type in which the outcome is most apt to be favorable. It may therefore serve as the starting point for a consideration of the causes and of the significance of such disturbances.

Causative Factors

1. Heredity. We may notice first of all that Albert's heredity is extremely bad. This, however, is by no means true of the group as a whole. Out of 159 cases on which information was available there was evidence of psychopathic inheritance in 46, that is, in 29 per cent. Of these 18 had parents who were mentally ill, seven had psychotic brothers and sisters and 21 more remote relatives. In 11 cases there was an alcoholic father. Albert's case was the only one in which both parents were alcoholic. In 101 cases there was no record of nervous and mental disorder. It would be too much to assume that the absence of any mention of neurotic relatives meant freedom from psychopathic taint, but it does seem safe to say that while the group as a whole had more than its share of bad inheritance, the family history in the majority of cases was as good as the average.

2. *Early Influences.* Unfavorable environmental influences were potent factors in this case. A survey of our cases indicates that such factors are more in evidence in the group as a whole than is bad heredity. Environmental maladjustments are mentioned in 64 per cent of the cases. We find 10 cases in which one of the parents had died during the patient's childhood and three cases in which both parents had died, two cases in which there is mention of quarreling and dissension in the home, and seven in which an overdominant and oversolicitous mother appears in the record. There were 19 cases in which the economic status is given as submarginal. Here again it must not be assumed that the absence of any mention of maladjustments in the case record means that the home environment was good. It follows therefore that unfavorable environmental influences were operative in a large number of our cases. At the same time we find not a few cases in which environmental influences seem considerably better than the average.

3. *Intelligence.* According to the Stanford-Binet test, Albert had a mental age of 14 years and 6 months. His rating is therefore above the average.[4] For the group as a whole the rating is probably somewhat below the average level. But it is not easy to judge. In 58 of our cases no ratings at all were secured because of the apathy or distractibility or antagonistic attitude of the patient. Those records which were secured are moreover merely minimums. Of those who took the test 37 scored below 10 years, 41 between 10 and 14 years, and 40 had mental ages of more than 14 years. It is not without significance that the two patients who made the highest score with mental ages of approximately 19 years are among the most hopelessly and bizarrely deluded. On

---

[4] If we take 14 years as the norm. Cf. F. L. Wells, *Mental Tests in Clinical Practice* (Yonkers, World Book Co., 1932), pp. 57–8.

the other hand all the cases of social recovery had at least average intelligence. Apparently the more intelligent and better educated individuals stand a better chance of finding their way out, but feeling more keenly and speculating more daringly, they may use their intelligence to build up elaborate delusional malformations.

4. Health. Albert W. had a serious heart ailment. In this respect he stands pretty much alone. This is due in part to the fact that patients with gross organic disease were intentionally excluded from the group. But the question did not arise in many cases and it seems safe to say that while the percentage of physical disease is greater in cases of dementia praecox than in a group of normal persons of the same age it is by no means characteristic. The heart ailment seems to have had little to do with Albert's mental difficulties.

Progress reports on the neuro-endocrine findings have been made elsewhere by those in charge of the research project. For the purpose of this study it is sufficient to say that while more endocrine dysfunction has been revealed than would be found in a group of normal persons, no single metabolic deviation has as yet been found to be characteristic either of dementia praecox as a group or of its several types.[5] An inspection of our cases indicates moreover that in quite a number of patients the endocrine dysfunction was corrected without any appreciable effect upon the mental condition and that in a few cases the mental condition cleared up without any alteration of the endocrine condition. This does not mean that these physiological factors were unimportant. There were other cases, not a few, in which the correcting of the endocrine dysfunction and the physical renovation had marked mental effects. It merely emphasizes the complexity of the problem. We do well to recognize the multiplicity of the causative factors and to proceed on the theory that if in any place

[5] Cf. Hoskins, " An Analysis of Schizophrenia from the Standpoint of the Investigator." *Journal of the American Medical Association*, 1931, vol. 97, p. 682.
Also: Hoskins and Jellinek, " The Schizophrenic Personality with Special Reference to Psychologic and Organic Concomitants." *Proceedings of the Association for Research in Nervous and Mental Disease*, vol. 14, Dec., 1933.

we can break the intricate chain of cause and effect we may enable the patient to come back.

5. *Life Situation.* The striking thing in the case of Albert W. is to be found in the powerful urge toward something better which led this poor handicapped waif to devote himself to long hours of serious reading and thinking, and in his picture of himself as represented by the term " apostogalia," which he had coined from the Greek. He wanted something. He had certain ideals or stand- ards by which he judged himself and his attainments. These standards, as I shall show in a later chapter, are functions of one's social relations. Any attempt to understand him would then re- quire a careful consideration of the group to which he belonged and of his adjustment to it.

(a) Social Relations. In Albert W. we see a boy with no parents worthy of the name. Those parents were taken away from him and never afterward did he succeed in finding another home. And yet we find this boy idealizing his parents. Perhaps the very lack of that which others possessed served to increase the sense of need, while the absence of disillusioning close contacts made possible the idealization. Later on in his remarkable interest in serious reading, developed probably through his association with the radicals he met on the road, we see him attempting to enter into association with the world's best and greatest minds. Mean- while his actual social adjustments were most unsatisfactory. He was a homeless wanderer who had lost caste even with his as- sociates on the road by turning " scab." Nevertheless he was one of those who are seeking to grow into something better than the standards represented by his early guides. It seems to have been this effort at growth which created the conflict.

In our general group we find that there are six cases in which there seems to have been an unsuccessful attempt to get away from the sense of personal failure by shifting the group loyalties and associating with bad companions. The great majority however have never questioned the implanted loyalties but have fallen far short in their performance. Most of them moreover take their shortcomings so seriously that they cannot bring themselves to acknowledge them to anyone else. The result is a sense of isolation and guilt which acts as a barrier between the individual and his fellows. We thus find 99 individuals of the retiring sort with few friends and few social contacts. Only 11 were said to have had many friends. Eighty-four of the group seemed to have a preference for solitary games and recreations. Fifty-six might be said to have been respected or accepted by their associates, 18 " razzed," and 58 ignored. The rest were classed as not clear. Judging objectively, we find seven cases in which the social adjustments may be rated as good, 34 average, 98 unsatisfactory and the rest not clear. The great majority had thus before their illness been maladapted to their external social environment and all, with six possible exceptions, were of those who in the light of their accepted ideals were subject to a serious sense of inner disharmony and isolation.

(b) Sex Adjustments. Albert was frank in discussing his sex maladjustments and it is certain that he had plenty of them. Even though the implanted standards could scarcely have been very high, he states that he worried much over the problem of auto-erotism, also that he fought against his homosexual tendencies and sought to " readjust his moral code." He speaks also of his sex morals as having descended to " the x y level." It is to be noted that he had nevertheless, according to his account, been capable of a genuine love affair, something which in this group is not over-frequent. This may be taken to represent the earnest seeking after something better which seems to characterize him.

In the group as a whole sex maladjustments appear clearly in the great majority of our cases. Of the 145 unmarried men 62 do not admit sex indulgence in any form. With hardly an exception these are individuals of the shut-in type who find insuperable difficulty in talking on this subject and are described by their friends as taking no interest in girls. Thirty-four admit or give evidence of difficulty with masturbation, 10 with erotic phantasy and 30 with both. Forty-three of the unmarried men admit heterosexual experiences which in three cases were marked by sexual impotence. Fifteen admit or give evidence of homosexual tendencies. Of the 30 married men 13 admit no difficulties in their sex adjustments. In four cases there is evidence of sexual impotence; three are divorced, three estranged from their wives, one is widowed and in two cases the wives are insane; 12 acknowledged extramarital relations and nine continued difficulty with masturbation and erotic phantasy. It would of course be absurd to assume that because a man did not acknowledge difficulty in managing the sex drive he was necessarily maladjusted sexually, and then go on to assume that those things which he did acknowledge were potent causative factors. Nevertheless a review of these cases leaves the definite impression that with the doubtful exception of a few married men there were none in the group who had arrived at healthy adult sexual development with wholesome expression of the sex drive. For all of them the realm of sex had apparently remained something at once terrifying and fascinating, something unassimilated in the organization of their experience and thus the source of much distress and discomfort.

(c) Vocational Adjustments. Albert tells us that at the time his disturbance began he had a good job. He had indeed no great reason to be satisfied with his vocational self-expression, but vocational thwarting does not seem in this case to be an immediate factor.

In our group of cases there were 26 in which the vocational situation would be regarded as definitely satisfactory and 56 in which it seemed equal to the average. In 90 cases the vocational adjustments were clearly unsatisfactory. Among the cases we find 95 unskilled workmen and 64 whose occupations required skill or training. We find six with incomes of $40 a week or more, 61 with incomes between $20 and $40, 77 under $20 and 29 without any income at all. We find 78 who had relatively stable employment, 56 who had made frequent changes and 20 who had been for some time out of work.

Summary. We may say in general that the 173 persons in this dementia praecox group are a somewhat handicapped lot. They have more than their share of hereditary taint; they have had considerably more than their share of unfavorable environmental influences; while seldom feeble-minded, they are somewhat below par intellectually; physically they are a trifle undersized and have less drive and vigor than a group of normal men of the same age. They are somewhat more subject to diseases of the flesh and about two-thirds of the patients presented evidences of one sort or another suggestive of endocrine deficiency. But in all this there is nothing distinctive of the group. In more than half of the cases the heredity seems at least no worse than the average. There is indeed a heavy burden of unfavorable environmental factors, but in quite a few cases the environmental factors are distinctly good. Intellectually some of these individuals rate high, and high ratings are often found in conjunction with bizarre delusions.

Maladjustments in the life situation, on the other hand, seem to be common to the entire group. There are scarcely any who have not some manifest maladjustments in one or more of the major fields of self-expression. We find none of whom it may be said with any certainty that he has attained to normal adult sexual development or to wholesome expression of the sex drive; in more than half of the cases there were clear vocational maladjustments and in two-thirds of them manifest social maladjustments were found. In 36 per cent of the cases we find clear maladjustments in all three fields and in 75 per cent in at least two fields. We may therefore conclude that in this group we have individuals who are thwarted in their effort to attain their major objectives in life in terms of their own picture of themselves. Anything therefore which might contribute to such a sense of failure and thwarting, whether it be poor intellectual or physical endowment, unfavorable influences, or maladjustments in the life situation would be a causative factor. But it cannot be too strongly emphasized that there is no objective measure of such maladjustments. The individual himself is the judge. The significant question from the standpoint of our particular problem is how the situation looks from the point of view of the individual himself.

The Reaction Patterns

The examination of the causative factors in dementia praecox has led us to the conclusion that the primary evil lies in the realm of social relationships, particularly in a life situation involving the sense of personal failure. We have found one characteristic common to the group as a whole: they are isolated from their fellows through a social judgment which either consciously or subconsciously they accept and pronounce upon themselves. In this they are to be contrasted sharply with the criminal and delinquent types. Such types are likewise social failures as judged by the standards of the family and of organized society, but they refuse to accept that judgment. Instead they characteristically seek social validation in groups which have standards of their own and support each other in rebellious, antisocial attitudes. But the psychotic accepts the social judgments of the group in which he has been reared, and by the standards which his early guides have implanted he stands condemned. The result is an intolerable loss of self-respect. In our group of cases we may distinguish three chief methods of dealing with such a sense of personal failure.

1. Drifting. A considerable number make little or no resistance. They do not fight. They do not attempt to turn over a new leaf. They do not try to do anything about it. They merely shut their eyes and drift. Very commonly they resort to easy modes of satisfaction. They withdraw into a world of phantasy, often hastening the process by a resort to drink or to drugs. Eventually they reach the point where the dream world has become for them the real world. The drive for self-realization is thus short-circuited and the individual becomes more and more listless and ineffective and unable to take care of himself. He thus becomes so peculiar and so much of a burden on his family or friends that they find it necessary to have him committed to the hospital. Such patients seldom show any great emotional disturbance. They have no marked hallucinations and their ideation is not particularly bizarre. But they drift down toward dissolution and destruction.

2. Delusional Misinterpretation. There are many others who meet the threatening failure by trying to " save their face." They refuse to admit defeat or error and resort to distortion of belief in order to escape the sense of failure and guilt. Most of our beliefs, as Dr. Macfie Campbell points out,[6] grow out of the requirements of the life situation and represent attempts to meet the stresses of existence. In other words, they represent the attempts to organize our experience in such a way that we can go on living and functioning in the world of men. Most of our current beliefs are incorrect. In delusional misinterpretation of the psychotic type we see this process carried to such an extreme that the individual is isolated from his fellows. These delusions are many and varied but they generally center around the problem of the relationship of the individual to his environment. Even though a delusional system may separate an individual from his group and cause him to be looked upon as queer, it serves to keep him from going to pieces and enables him to maintain a certain degree of integration and poise.

3. Panic. But few individuals can drift down to destruction or succeed in building up an effective system of delusional misinterpretation without at some time becoming aware of their danger. The result is a greater or less degree of emotional disturbance. In its extreme form this emotional disturbance may appear as that profound despair and hopelessness in which the sufferer loses all interest either in the external world or in himself and he feels himself to be as one dead. It may also assume the form of acute upheaval as exemplified in the case of Albert W. Such a disturbance may occur either in the drifting or in the deluded types or in persons who have seemed fairly well adjusted. My own severe disturbance belonged in this particular reaction type and I am proceeding on the theory that it is to be sharply contrasted with the end results of personality disintegration or delusional malformation. Such disturbances, whether of the stuporous or agitated type, are not in themselves evils, but are analogous to fever or inflammation in the body. They are attempts at cure

[6] *Delusion and Belief* (Harvard University Press, 1926).

and reorganization which are closely related to certain recognized types of religious experience.

These general reaction types are easily recognized in their typical forms. But they usually occur in combination and it is no easy task to classify our cases according to the reaction patterns. Before making such an attempt it has seemed necessary to study carefully the characteristic ideation and behavior in order to discover, if possible, more objective criteria which will help us in placing particular cases.

Content of Thought

In the hospital to which I was sent as a patient little attention was paid to my ideas. It was assumed that such disorders were rooted in some as yet undiscovered organic factor and that the ideas were secondary or accidental. Such a view has been fairly common in the psychiatric world. The great advances have come however with the recognition of the tremendous significance to the patient of his ideas and emotions. They are to him reality, grim, terrifying, torturing, mocking, fascinating, and if we are to arrive at any true understanding of our patient and of the world in which he lives we must know what is on his mind. This is in fact the inner world which it is our task to explore.

1. The Sense of the Mysterious. Albert W.'s disturbance began with the idea that something strange was going on. He felt himself in possession of a power that he did not have before and he began to have a "flood of mental pictures as though an album within were unfolding itself." Then came the dark woman in a vision, whom he took to be supernatural. This is thoroughly characteristic of acute disturbances. They begin generally with some eruption of the subconscious which is interpreted as a manifestation of the supernatural. The impact of such an experience is apt to be terrific. It may destroy the foundations of the mental organization and upset the structure upon which the judgments and reasoning processes are based. We have then that bewildered state which is called "schizophrenia" or "dementia praecox." The sufferer finds himself in a strange new world in which previous experience and accepted standards of value do not apply. He sees strange meanings in everything about him and he is sure of only one thing, that things are not what they seem. The deeper levels of the mind are tapped and in many cases the mental processes are quickened. Ideas and pictures flash into the mind as if from an outside source and constitute the " voices " and " visions " which loom so large in psychiatric examinations. Very commonly it is as if the conscious self had descended to some lower region where it is no longer in control but at the mercy of the primitive and terrifying ideas and imagery which throng in upon it. The eyes are opened so that one seems to see back to the beginning of creation. One seems to have lived perhaps in many previous existences. Such ideas we find with striking frequency in case after case. To the individual concerned they carry conviction because they seem so utterly new, so completely apart from all his previous thinking and reading. Such observations are in line with Jung's conception of a " racial unconscious." In any case it is such a *regression* to a lower level of the mental life which is characteristic of these experiences. We seldom encounter any breaks in the memory chain or any such " splitting " of the personality as that which Morton Prince has described. For this reason the term " schizophrenia " which has been used to describe this condition as a substitute for the term " dementia praecox " seems a misnomer.

In 54 of our cases the onset was sudden and involved acute emotional disturbance. In 68 cases it was of the subacute type, the acute outbreak having been preceded by a somewhat protracted period of withdrawal or of delusion-building. In 51 cases the onset was insidious. In only seven cases were there any factors in the immediate life situation which might account for the mental disturbance. In practically all the cases the disturbance seemed explainable rather in terms of inner disharmony and conflict which had reached the stage in which a solution was inevitable. Among the cases with acute onset we find four in which the outcome was social recovery, and seven improvement. Among the cases with subacute onset there are three which resulted in social

recovery and three in improvement. In general the acute onset
with its marked sense of mystery tends to be associated with the
profounder types of disturbance, characterized by archaic symbolism, bizarre ideation, also by much religious concern and by
a relatively good recovery rate. (Cf. Chart I)

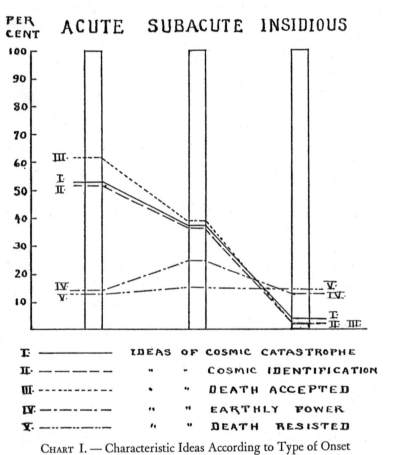

CHART I. — Characteristic Ideas According to Type of Onset

2. *The Sense of Peril.* The second step which we observed in
the development of Albert's psychosis was an acute sense of peril.
He thought he was going to die. Then he saw things in a new
light and he thought the " dawn of creation " had come. He was

living in a different world. Then it came to him that he had
lived before this present life and that he was a much more important person than he had ever dreamed. In a previous existence
he had been Jonah. He had also been Christ. Most of the time
he had been St. Augustine. It came to him that there was a great
" I and You contest " going on, a struggle for supremacy on the
part of certain groups, though in relation to this struggle it was
not clear where he stood.

Here we have a group of ideas which appear over and over
again in the profounder disturbances. In 57 of our cases we find
ideas of an impending world change of some sort and of great
issues at stake. In 53 cases we find in the patient exalted ideas as
to his own rôle. In 41 cases these two ideas are found in conjunction. One patient thus has the idea that the world is about
to fall to pieces and that he himself is the world. Three have
the idea that the world is about to be destroyed and that its fate
is entirely dependent upon them; if they die the world is ruined.
Three others have received revelations that the second coming of
Christ is about to take place and that they themselves are to have
a central rôle in this great event, presumably as the present-day
incarnation of the Christ spirit. Another announces that he is
to be crucified. Two speak of themselves as the " Son of God."
One man gets very much excited when questioned about his religion and announces belligerently that " little Charlie can lick
God." This patient has the besetting idea that it is getting very
cold and that the great ice age is coming. Another considers
himself a reincarnation of Abraham. Another is the devil and
he is greatly concerned lest all the Bibles be burned. Another is
alternately God and the devil.

As in the case of Albert it frequently happens that the rôles shift.
The individual is first one and then another personage and sometimes nothing at all. At one moment he may be a zero quantity
and at the next moment the Almighty. Twenty-three acknowledged that they had had such ideas, but refused to go into particulars. These seemed very sensitive on the subject. Ideas of
mission are found in 24 cases and ideas of rebirth in 23. These

ideas are seldom found except in conjunction with ideas of cosmic catastrophe and cosmic identification. Ideas of death, self-inflicted or accepted as inevitable, appear in 61 cases. Of this number, ideas of cosmic catastrophe appear also in only 36 and ideas of cosmic identification in 36. This may be accounted for by the fact to which Hoch and MacCurdy call attention, that ideas of death are characteristic of the deeply depressed and stuporous types, those who do not, like Albert W., go on to believe in some coming " dawn of creation " and a rôle which they can play, but remain fixed in the despair and gloom of the death idea. In such cases paucity of ideation is characteristic.[7] Deep depression, when characterized by self-blame and acceptance of responsibility, tends toward favorable outcomes. Although this fact cannot be clearly demonstrated on the basis of this group of cases alone, we are taking the ideas of death, together with the ideas of cosmic catastrophe and cosmic identification, as characteristic of the panic reactions of the profounder sort. It is to be noted however that ideas of death thought of as inflicted by enemies are not so likely to be accompanied by ideas of cosmic catastrophe and cosmic identification. Such ideas are generally associated with concealment reactions. So also are the ideas of self-importance, when these are limited to earthly power and influence and do not go on to assume cosmic or religious significance. Ideas of change of sex were found in seven cases distributed among all reaction types.

It is to be noted that the sense of peril as manifested in our cases applies almost equally to the self and to the world as a whole. There is little setting of the individual over against the world. A danger to himself is a danger to the entire world, and if there are enemies of the self they are enemies of the cosmic order also. The stuporous types, who are characterized by ideas of death without cosmic concern, may be those who are inclined to be self-depreciative. It may be that those who identify themselves with the cosmic and the divine are the egotists who find it difficult to get off the throne, but the evidence is not clear.

3. *The Sense of Personal Responsibility.* In going to the police,

---

[7] *Benign Stupors* (New York, Macmillan Co., 1921), pp. 191–2.

telling them of his court record and asking for an investigation of the supposed charges against him, Albert W. at the beginning of his disturbance showed a distinct desire to face the facts and a willingness to accept responsibility for his past actions. Throughout his disturbance and afterwards he showed remarkable frankness, telling apparently everything, even that which was damaging to his pride. It is also to be noted that in spite of his serious heart difficulty he kept on doing hard manual labor almost up to the time he was taken to the hospital. At the same time he had ideas of persecution. He thought that he was being talked about and that he was being hunted, he did not know for what. This is characteristic of the stormy phase of dementia praecox. All sorts of ideas are mixed up together in loose and unorganized form. Ideas of persecution appear even in such clear-cut attempts to face the situation and readiness to accept responsibility as we see in the case of Albert. We must not therefore attach too much importance to the mere occurrence of a persecutory idea. The question is always how far that idea represents a dominating trend in the patient's personality. 1532046

Of our 173 cases, 130 give evidence of the concealment reaction. This is to be found in four chief forms. The most frequent is that which may be termed EXTERNALIZATION OF CONSCIENCE. This is clear in 113 cases. In 73 of these the patient hears *accusing voices* which charge him with all sorts of improper behavior, or he may see people talking about him and laughing at him wherever he goes. In 22 cases the sense of guilt reveals itself in the idea that the *mind is being read* or the thoughts recorded by means of dictaphones and broadcast over the radio. In 14 cases there are ideas of being followed, usually by detectives or spies. Ideas of being *poisoned* or drugged are found in 37 cases and of being killed in 29 cases. These ideas may all be regarded as indications of a resisted and uneasy conscience.

TRANSFER OF BLAME is evident in 70 cases. *Electrical currents* shooting through the body, usually under the control of some enemy and playing upon the genitals, figure in 37 cases and may be looked upon as acceptable explanations of unacceptable physical cravings. *Hypnotic or other personal or super-personal influences* which control the mind are found in 32 cases, as explanations usually of unacceptable thoughts. *Circumvention of one's plans* through individuals or organized groups, usually secret societies, is found in 17 cases.

FICTITIOUS SELF-IMPORTANCE appears in a large number of cases. In 10 cases it is sufficiently powerful to enable the patient to effect a delusional reconstruction which permits him to keep on functioning with some degree of comfort. Where such a reconstruction is made on the religious basis it is commonly free from externalization of conscience and transfer of blame.

The INCAPACITATION reaction, in which physical illness is made to bear the responsibility for the personal failure, is found in 29 cases. While unquestionably a concealment device which seeks to save the individual's self-respect, it differs from the preceding reactions in that it involves the recognition of difficulty and it locates that difficulty within the individual. It is, however, a confession of weakness and a bid for sympathy and attention.

The acceptance of responsibility with the reaction of SELF-BLAME is found in 19 cases. It may be noted that in three of these there has been social recovery; in three, sufficient improvement to be sent back into the community; and in five others, a temporary recovery.

4. Erotic Involvement. Throughout his disturbed period Albert W. was little concerned about sex. He was occupied instead with religion and with cosmic affairs. But the problem of sex had figured in his previous history and it became a complicating factor after the stormy period of his second disturbance had passed. Some obscene drawings for which he was responsible led to his discharge from an occupational therapy class and thus denied to him one of the important sources of help.

As already indicated, the sex factor figures in a large proportion of our cases. In many cases that which is at stake is the preservation of the integrity of the individual against the disintegrating power of the primitive cravings. Threatened by instinctual claims no longer capable of being satisfied in the present stage of development, the sufferer is unable either to renounce them or to control them.[8] Like Laocoön in the old Greek statue he is being overwhelmed by the reptilian monsters of sex. Not a few talk frankly of the fearful and disgusting, yet fascinating, imagery which swarms in upon them, supposedly at the behest of hostile forces. It is probable that the patient who is hearing himself charged with sodomy and incest and other awful things is merely telling us in a roundabout way that he is being assailed by such ideas. It must be clearly recognized, as Alexander points out (*Ibid.,* p. 82), that for such sufferers ideas have the value of actions. They are for them reality.

Of the entire group of cases, 36 had so far lost their self-respect as to indulge openly in erotic manifestations. Of these, 16 had passed through a panic reaction and 13 belonged in the drifting group. Only seven were found among the 81 cases showing the concealment reaction. Fifty-six patients displayed no open eroticism but acknowledged more or less frankly their difficulties in managing the sex drive. In the remaining 81 cases there was no direct evidence and the patients themselves were reticent in discussing the matter. Of the 36 who displayed open eroticism there are three who are now at home (Chart II) but of these only one, a man who had at the same time a pronounced self-accusatory attitude, can be said to be really improved. Of those who have been reticent or evasive concerning their sex problems and who have succeeded in keeping within the limits of decent behavior, one is rated as a social recovery, eight are improved and out of the hospital, while six are slightly improved and out of the hospital.

These figures support the view that the primary evil in a large proportion of the cases is the short-circuiting of the urge for self-realization and the dissolution of the personality under the influence of instinctual cravings which have got beyond control, and that this occurs most surely in those cases in which the individual makes no resistance. They show furthermore that the preservation of the appearance of decency through the seclusive, evasive,

[8] Cf. Alexander, *Psychoanalysis of the Total Personality* (Washington, Nervous and Mental Disease Publishing Co., 1930), Lecture V.

reticent attitudes tends to prevent the more extreme forms of disintegration and that such individuals may even get better and go
out. They also show the therapeutic value of confession, and they

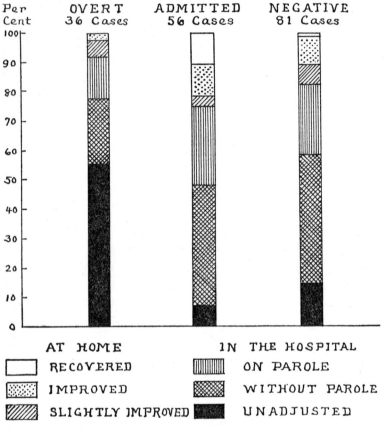

CHART II. — Present Condition in Relation to Erotic Involvement

indicate that self-blame, even to the point of morbidity, may not
be in itself an evil but an attempt at cure which makes or breaks
the sufferer.

CLINICAL TYPES AND CLINICAL RESULTS

The hypothesis upon which we are proceeding is that the primary evil in dementia praecox lies in the realm of social rela-

tionship, particularly in a life situation involving the sense of personal failure, and that the common clinical pictures are determined by the various reaction patterns which have been employed to meet such situations. We have assumed furthermore that in the psychotic types the sense of failure is either consciously or subconsciously accepted and that the major reaction patterns consist of drifting, concealment and panic. We are now in position to group our cases in accordance with the dominant reaction patterns which are in evidence. We shall then be able to check them with the clinical groupings made by the hospital staff and to draw certain conclusions in regard to the clinical significance of the various reaction types.

The study which has been made of the content of thought leads to the following conclusions which will be helpful in classifying our cases:

1. The presence of ideas of death, of cosmic catastrophe, or of cosmic identification may be taken as the mark of the profounder panic reactions. The ideas of cosmic catastrophe and cosmic identification tend to occur together as part of a constellation of ideas which includes also ideas of rebirth, previous existence, mission, and so forth. Ideas of death, when accepted and not resisted as due to enemies, occur also in this same constellation. The presence of any one of these ideas means that others of this constellation are likely also to be present. It may furthermore be taken to indicate that the sufferer has experienced one of those profound regressions which represents a journey to the lower regions, that grim wilderness of the lost which we are seeking to explore.

2. While the concealment reactions are also marked by certain characteristic ideas representing the externalization of conscience, transfer of blame, fictitious self-importance and incapacitation, the classifications must be made more upon the basis of dominant mood and attitude rather than upon that of sporadic ideas which may at one time or another be expressed.

3. The drifting type is characterized not merely by the absence of the positive findings listed under 1 and 2, but also by the lack of the fighting spirit in the face of difficulties.

4. An acute onset implies the absence in their advanced stages of the character tendencies described under 2 and 3 and indicates a panic reaction free from the more malignant complications.

1. The Drifters. Thirty-five cases are characterized by the lack of any fighting spirit. Of these, 17 show sporadic concealment reactions; 13 hear accusing voices; three have ideas of being killed; four show the tendency to transfer blame in ideas of hypnosis and electrical currents; and one shows a marked incapacitation reaction. Three of the group did fairly well in their studies at school and six had passable vocational records, but the group as a whole was of the shiftless ne'er-do-well type who never make good in anything. Most of them are of the well-meaning, passively good variety, lacking in drive and determination. All are of the type who drift unresistingly down toward dissolution and destruction, often without any attempt to keep up appearances or to maintain self-respect.

2. The Self-Deceivers. Thirty-nine cases present a sharp contrast to the first group in that they make a real effort to keep up outward appearances. They are of those that refuse to admit defeat and error and they give evidence of some real fighting spirit. Three have been successful vocationally and 13 fairly successful. Among them we find plentifully represented evidences of the repressed conscience and of attempts to shift responsibility. The important characteristic in most of the cases is the surly, sulky, fault-finding, suspicious attitudes which have become more or less dominant.

3. The Panic-Stricken. The remaining 99 cases give evidence of the profounder sort of disturbance as indicated by ideas of death, cosmic catastrophe, or cosmic identification. Among these we may distinguish two types, those in whom the panic or upheaval takes place in an individual whose habitual reaction is that of suppression of conscience and transfer of blame, and those in whom there are no such complications.

(a) Simple Types. There are 57 cases in which the panic states are relatively free from the various concealment devices and in which the concealment reactions, when they do occur, are transitory. These individuals are all fairly free from the tendency to sulk and find fault and dwell on their grievances. With a few exceptions the disturbance began with a sudden onset. Of these 57 cases, 12 had good vocational records and 24 fair. This group

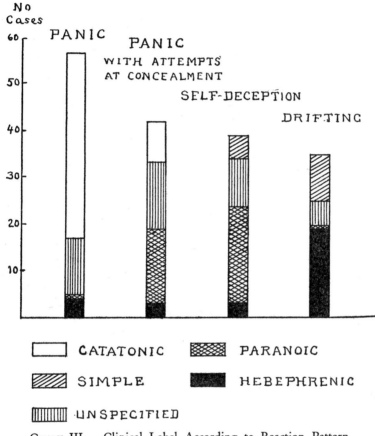

CHART III.—Clinical Label According to Reaction Pattern

likewise includes a relatively large proportion of the pleasant, likable type that are accepted and respected by their associates.

(b) Mixed Types. Forty-two cases are of those in whom the panic reaction takes place in a personality already considerably warped through its efforts to interpret the life situation in terms favorable to self-respect. In general make-up this group is very similar to the self-deceived. They are of those who find it hard to admit defeat or error. Vocationally the figures on these two groups are almost identical. Of the 42 individuals in this group four have good records, 13 fair and 25 poor.

4. *Reaction Types and Psychiatric Labels.* Chart III shows the psychiatric labels as determined at the regular medical staff meetings of the research service when distributed according to the above reaction types. It will be seen that the correlation is close, especially so in the case of the catatonic and panic types. The differences are for the most part due to the fact that in the grouping according to reaction pattern no categories were made corresponding to " unspecified " and none to those end results designated by the term " hebephrenic." The five cases of " simple dementia praecox " in the concealment group are accounted for by the greater emphasis placed upon dominant attitudes as compared with sporadic delusional formations.

5. *Reaction Types and Outcome.* Chart IV shows the present condition of the patients in the four groups. The seven " social recoveries " are those who have been out of the hospital for a year or more, who have proved themselves able and willing to work and to get along with their families and friends, and who seem free from psychotic beliefs and attitudes. The 14 who are out of the hospital " improved " are those who have shown marked improvement in their ability and willingness to work and get along with their associates but who have not been out of the hospital for more than a year or who are still clinging to some of their psychotic beliefs and attitudes. The 11 " slightly improved " are those who, while somewhat better, have been able to go home chiefly by virtue of the devotion and forbearance of their families. Of those in the hospital 39 are " on parole." This means that they have proved themselves able to work and obey the rules sufficiently to be trusted with the freedom of the grounds. The 62 " without parole " are those who are able to keep themselves moderately neat, to do at least some simple work and to take part in the recreational activities, but who have not yet proved

their right to the freedom of the grounds. The 40 patients in the
" unadjusted group " are those who are non-co-operative, shiftless, careless of personal appearance, mute, resistive or otherwise
disturbed.[9]

It is to be noted that all of the cases of social recovery and all
but two of those classed as " improved " are to be found in cases
characterized by the panic reaction. It is also to be noted that of
the 40 unadjusted patients all but eight are to be found in the
drifting group or else in the panic group, simple type. *We may
thus see in the drifting reaction type a marked tendency toward
deterioration* even in the face of the unremitting therapeutic efforts of the research service. We may also observe *the stabilizing
effect of delusional misinterpretation.* In both groups characterized by the concealment reaction we find only two social recoveries
and only three who are classed as improved. We also find only
eight who are rated as unadjusted, and inspection of these eight
cases reveals that they are just across the border. *Most striking
is the tendency of the panic reaction to produce change either for
the better or for the worse. Not only do we find the largest proportion of social recoveries and of improvements in the panic
group, but we also observe that when panic occurs in the warped
personality it may serve to break up the shell of delusional misinterpretation and set the victim free.* We thus find two in this latter
group who have made social recoveries and three who are mark-
edly improved. We observe also that 19 of the panic group are
classed as unadjusted. And these figures do not tell the whole
story, for among those of the panic group who are now rated as

---

[9] This grouping follows in the main the ratings of the research service as given
out in September, 1931, and described by Drs. Erickson and Hoskins in the *American
Journal of Psychiatry* for July, 1931. It differs from this classification in that it distinguishes three groups among those now at home, a task that required a visit to each
of the discharged patients. Classes E and F are moreover thrown together and four
patients who had been placed in Class D chiefly because they had shown some improvement and needed encouragement were counted among the " unadjusted."

Six of the patients included in the 173 have died. Two of these committed suicide,
one after escaping from the hospital and the other after being sent home as " improved."
Both of these were classed as " out of the hospital, unimproved." The others died in the
hospital. Two of these belonged in the unadjusted group and were steadily growing
worse. The others had made an institutional adjustment. One of them had a parole.

unadjusted are six who have been out of the hospital, rated in five cases as social recoveries.

6. *Fifteen Cases of Social Recovery.* Of our 173 cases there were only seven who had finished their year of probation, had

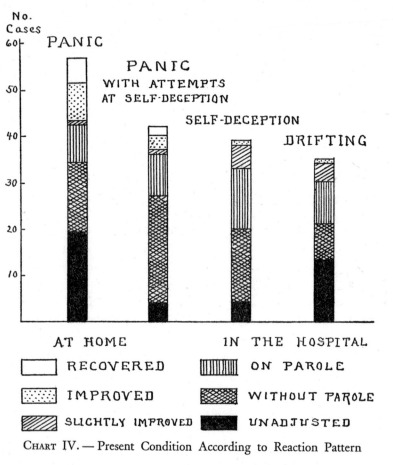

CHART IV. — Present Condition According to Reaction Pattern

demonstrated their ability and willingness to work and to get along with their family and friends, and who seemed free from psychotic ideas and attitudes. For purposes of comparison it has therefore seemed expedient to supplement this group by the addition of eight cases not in the research group, with whom I have myself done intensive work.[10] This gives a total of 15 cases of social recovery — not a large number, but it may enable us to arrive at some generalizations regarding the factors which make for recovery.

What strikes one first of all in looking over this group is their relatively good equipment and their relatively favorable life situation. While the research group as a whole is somewhat handicapped, somewhat below par intellectually, a trifle undersized and deficient in drive and vigor, we have in these 15 cases of social recovery individuals of more than average intelligence and vigor. And whereas in the research group as a whole, 75 per cent are blocked in at least two of the major fields of self-expression and 36 per cent in all three fields, we find in these social recoveries none who are blocked in all three fields and only 33 per cent who are blocked in more than one. In nine of the 15 cases the vocational adjustments were good and in the others they were fair. Two had incomes of more than $40 a week, 10 between $20 and $40, two were students with excellent records and one an efficient housekeeper with a good bank account acquired under difficulties. All but one had stable employment. Seven of the 15 were married and six of these had children. Eleven of them talked with more or less frankness of their sex problems, recognizing these as the source of their difficulties. Although in some cases of the " shut-in " type, all were of the sort that make a good impression and are accepted and generally respected by their associates. All of them, in other words, were good material and they had something to come back to.

We are also struck by certain characteristics of their psychotic experiences. In 10 cases the onset was quite sudden and the disturbance very acute. Of the remaining cases, four became acutely disturbed following a period of seclusiveness and suspiciousness of the paranoic type. Thirteen of the 15 gave clear expression to the ideas which this study has shown to be characteristic of

[10] During my period of service at Worcester I wrote up and interviewed more or less systematically some 35 patients in addition to those in the research group. These 8 cases include all those of the schizophrenic type in which the outcome was social recovery.

profound panic and upheaval. Of these all showed religious concern with appropriate mood and attitude and freedom from
facetiousness and silliness and ugliness of temper. Of the two
remaining cases, one showed marked religious concern and worry
over his sins, while the other talked of his difficulties with remarkable frankness and intelligence. It may also be noted that
of the 15 cases all but three remained in the hospital less than one
year.

It is clear that in the case of individuals such as these, with
good equipment and favorable life situations, it may be possible
for them to resume their places in society even though they may
be impaired as a result of their psychosis. In two there is evidence
of such impairment, due chiefly to discouragement and lack of
understanding on the part of friends. In three cases there has
been more than one disturbed period. But even these individuals
seem none the worse for the experience. In three cases there is
evidence that the psychosis has served to clear up problems which
for some years had been obstructing the normal functioning and
development.

One of these cases was an attractive, vigorous man with a good
industrial record who had begun to drink heavily and developed
some marked paranoid tendencies. He thought the lodges were
after him and that enemies were on his trail. He even went to
the police and asked permission to carry a gun in order to pro-
tect himself. Shortly after this he went to his wife and confessed
to her the marital infidelities and sexual irregularities which had
been preying on his mind. This confession she accepted in good
part. With this the picture changed from a malignant to a benign one. He became indeed much more disturbed emotionally
and it became necessary to send him to the hospital. But he
ceased to be concerned about his enemies. Instead he began to
blame himself and to worry for fear something was going to
happen to his wife. After several months of severe disturbance
his mind cleared and he has now for four years been out of the
hospital. According to the latest reports he seems to be better
and his home life is happier than it has ever been before.

Another case was that of a tall, vigorous, attractive and capable woman who against the protests of her friends married a man who proved to be both alcoholic and paranoic. A few years after their marriage he had to be taken to a state hospital. But she left him there only a short time. She had been brought up to believe that a wife should be true to her husband through thick and thin. Besides that she was not ready to admit to her friends that they had been right. She therefore took him out against the advice of the physicians at the hospital and kept him out for twenty years, all the time queerer and more difficult to live with. They could not even sit down to the table but that he saw some sinister meaning in the way she had arranged the knives and forks and glasses or placed the chairs. She began at length to develop paranoic ideas of her own. She thought people were following her and talking about her. Then came the death of her mother and a visit back to her old home in Sweden. After her return there came a profound disturbance. She became stuporous and had to be tube-fed. For four long years she remained in the back wards of the hospital under the label of " dementia praecox, catatonic type, very much demented." She then cleared up and has now for five years been out of the hospital. Her husband, deprived of her protection, had meanwhile found his way to an institution and she is now free of the impossible situation which his presence had created. But even before her release her dominant feeling was that she had found a new lease on life.

In another case, a young man of good intelligence and fair education had been addicted to the practice of masturbation from his fourth year on. As a child he had had night terrors, was subject to melancholy spells and had worried continually about his health. He talked to no one of his inner difficulties and was seclusive and shy. In his nineteenth year he developed definite paranoic tendencies. Wherever he went he thought he was being watched. This difficulty did not develop to the point of acute disturbance. He was brought to the hospital and there talked over his difficulties with remarkable frankness and intelligence.

There is reason to believe that he has now in large measure found the solution to his problem.

RELIGIOUS CONCERN

The most striking feature in the case of Albert W. is to be found in its religious aspects and their implications. All through his first disturbance he was tremendously concerned about the problems of life and death, of survival and destruction, and about his relationship to that which was supreme in his hierarchy of loyalties. For a time he thought he was dead and in hell, and in himself he saw diabolical features. Then he was translated into heaven. The trees took on a magnificent appearance. He recognized the work of the supernatural and he thought that the dawn of creation had come. He studied the formation of the clouds and the sky took on for him an appearance wonderful beyond expression. He heard an infinite voice say that six o'clock was the appointed time for the arrival of God's decrees. He visualized himself as passing from an earthly to a spiritual life and from the red to the white. At one time he felt a light within him as though he had touched the Holy Grail. He identified himself with Jesus, with Augustine, with the martyrs of old. It came to him that the second coming of the Lord was at hand and that in this he himself was to have a most important rôle to play. He also suffered severe reactions. He was tempted to injure others and he thought of himself as Judas, as Jonah, and even as the devil. He states that before his disorder he wanted to be the same religious person he had been when he was a child and that his disturbance brought him proof that there is such a thing as a spiritual type. He felt that through his disturbance he had found new life and new purpose.

Albert's story, as he told it before the staff and later before a group of students, abounded in rare flashes of insight and in its simplicity, and at times beauty of language, it bore the stamp of genuineness. It seemed the story of one who had been through a great spiritual adventure. His attitude may therefore be taken as representing a high degree of religious concern. In this experience which he describes we may see the better part of himself seeking to break through and take possession. For seven years he had been a divided personality. On the one hand there were the tendencies which had made him such a problem to the Division of Child Guardianship; which had landed him in the reform school, and which had then sent him forth into his unsatisfactory roving existence. On the other hand, there was the desire for fellowship with the world's best and greatest minds which had been expressing itself in his long course of serious reading. These two tendencies could not exist forever side by side. He could not continue to worship both God and mammon. One or the other had to become ascendant. The disturbance seems to represent the attempt to solve that inner conflict and to bring about a state of equilibrium between the contending forces. Thus in its inner meaning Albert's experience had profound religious significance. This religious urge revealed itself moreover in appropriate and consistent form. He was absorbed in the problem of reality and of his relation to it. His mood swung from despair to ecstasy or from ecstasy to despair and seemed to be quite in keeping with the situation in which he felt himself. And from this disturbed period he emerged with the feeling that he had passed from an earthly to something in the nature of a spiritual life. In other words he himself interpreted it in religious terms.

It has been shown that this concern with the problem of ultimate reality is characteristic of a large proportion of our cases and that the ideas we find in Albert W. are common to experiences of this type. We may assume that the presence of ideas of cosmic catastrophe and of cosmic identification, wherever we find them, indicate something of this same experience, and when along with these ideas there are appropriate mood and attitude, and when the patient has recourse to prayer, attends religious services or performs religious acts, we may say that he shows *marked religious concern.* So also when there are ideas of death and the mood is one of despair and worry over one's sins. When however such ideas and moods are transient, when the mood and attitude during the stormy period are often inappropriate, when there are streaks of facetiousness and spells of surliness, we may rate the *religious concern* as *moderate* and question the extent to which the religious concern is likely to take possession. Patients who show none of these ideas and attitudes, who do not attend the services or observe any of the common religious forms, are to be rated as *without religious concern.*

Albert's statement that he wanted to become again the same religious person he had been when he was a child must be taken with a good deal of allowance. In the light of his general record we may conclude that he was reading his present interests back into the past and thus creating for himself an imaginary golden age. His record is certainly a bad one. He was unruly, dishonest and sexually maladjusted. But there was apparently a tendency to idealize his worthless parents even during his unhappy childhood. Then came the long course of serious reading which, even though there may have been no interest in formal religion, seems to place him *during the pre-psychotic period* in the group of the moderately religious. By that is meant that there seems to have been some conscious seeking after the fellowship of the best even though the life he was living was very inconsistent with that desire.

Among our cases are six individuals who seem to have identified themselves with antisocial groups. They are said to have associated by preference with " toughs " and were apparently not ashamed to be called " bad boys." One of these, a boy with a record of stealing and general toughness, developed an acute disturbance. The rest showed no sense of guilt or worry but drifted aimlessly and unresistingly down toward dissolution.

Sixty-eight of our cases, so far as the fragmentary early histories permit us to judge, are individuals who have never shown any particular religious interest. They have not gone to church or displayed any signs of religious concern. There are no indications however that they have ever identified themselves with antisocial groups. They seem to be of the great multitude who passively accept the ideals and teachings of their early guides without attempting to do much about them. If questioned about their religious beliefs they would probably say that of course they believed in God. It would be equally probable that they would show signs of discomfort and seek to change the subject. Of these two groups, 74 cases in all, we say of their pre-psychotic life that *religious concern was not evident*.

Eighty-nine are of those who not merely accept the teachings of their early guides but attempt also to do something about them. They go to church or to mass or to synagogue. They may even perform certain private devotional acts. But their religion remains on the whole rather formal and superficial. Of these we say that their *religious concern was moderate*.

Ten are individuals who have taken their religion much more seriously. One of these was a clergyman, one a theological student, two were planning to study for the ministry, two were zealous church workers and four were for a time ardent members of holiness sects. Of these we say that their *religious concern was marked*.

In going through the case records, one is not infrequently struck with the evidences of fluctuation in religious interest. We find in some histories that shortly before the onset the patient began to display great interest in religion. He would spend much time in prayer or reading the Bible or attending religious services, where before he had been rather indifferent. In other cases we read that some months before his commitment the patient stopped going to church and lost all interest in religion. Chart V shows the cases rated as to religious concern and distributed according to reaction pattern both before and at the time of onset. This chart brings out strikingly the accentuation of religious concern at the time of onset in the panic reactions and its diminution in the concealment and drifting reactions.

We thus find added support for the view that religious concern tends to appear wherever men are seeking to face their difficulties and are trying to become better. These findings are in line with Professor Wieman's definition of religion as " man's acute awareness of the realm of unattained possibility and the behavior which results from this awareness." [11]

[11] *The Wrestle of Religion with Truth* (New York, Macmillan Co., 1927), p. 135.

In nine of our cases religion is a factor in the delusional reconstruction which has taken place, in three of these to a very pronounced degree. In fifteen cases we have something of a delusional reconstruction without any apparent religious motivation.

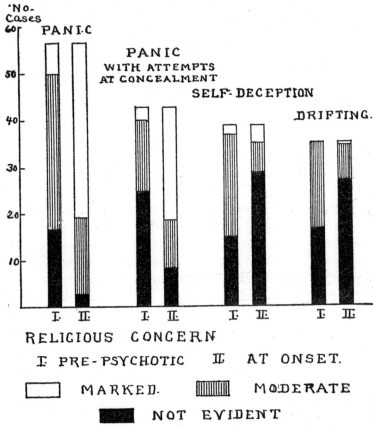

CHART V. — Religious Concern According to Reaction Pattern

In the latter group are ten cases characterized by bitter, suspicious, fault-finding, non-co-operative attitudes. These antisocial attitudes are absent in the first group. With two partial exceptions the patients in the first group are friendly and co-operative. This is particularly true of the three cases in which the religious motivation was pronounced.

The conclusion follows that religion is not an " escape from reality." On the contrary it represents an attempt to deal with those loyalties and values which are regarded as ultimate. Where it does figure in a delusional reconstruction it tends to produce an interpretation of the life situation which is socially acceptable as compared with the bitter and antisocial attitudes found in the other paranoid types. Religion, as I shall show in a later chapter, is an attempt to raise one's values to the level of the cosmic or universal and to establish and maintain right relationship with those to whom one looks for response and approval, those whose composite impress is represented in the idea of God.

Nature's Power to Heal

This survey of the wilderness of the lost tends to support the hypothesis with which we started, that many of the more serious psychoses are essentially problem-solving experiences which are closely related to certain types of religious experience. We have seen that my own experience is by no means an isolated one. Those strange ideas that came to me, ideas of world catastrophe, of death, of rebirth, of cosmic importance and of mission, are found in case after case. They tend to occur in conjunction with one another. Where we find one we are apt to find the others also, and the presence of one of these ideas, in so far as it is autochthonous and not derived from other persons, is sufficient to establish the presumption that the individual concerned has made this grim journey to the lower regions and has stood face to face with the great realities of death and life.

We have also discovered that such ideas are not to be found in all cases but only in those who are trying to face their difficulties. In many of our cases such an attempt was hardly in evidence and the symptoms which brought the patient to the hospital represented the end results of certain malignant character tendencies. In some of these the urge for self-realization had become short-circuited so that the unhappy individual was left isolated from his fellows and shut off from his real objectives in life. In other cases the sufferer sought to escape from the intolerable sense of personal failure by misinterpreting the situation and resorting to such devices as fault-finding, making excuses, blaming others, magnifying his own importance, and the like. Among the cases representing the reactions of drifting and concealment we found little religious concern and almost no recoveries. In the drifting reaction the tendency was uniformly in the direction of disintegration; in the concealment reaction it was toward arrested development and stabilization on an unsatisfactory basis. Few of those who had worked out a delusional system went all to pieces and few of them recovered. Against these end results of malignant character tendencies we see standing out in sharp contrast the acute disturbances which represent the attempt to face the realities of a difficult life situation. Among these cases there were not a few recoveries. There were also many who went to the back wards and stayed there. The acute upheaval or panic reaction thus tends either to make or to break. We may therefore draw the conclusion that such disturbances are not necessarily evils but, like fever or inflammation in the physical organism, they are attempts by regression to the lower levels of mental life to assimilate certain hitherto unassimilated masses of life experience. They represent the deliquescence of the old sets and attitudes which make possible new formations. They are essentially purposive; in this group we even found individuals whose lives had been changed for the better.

This interpretation means that in the ailments of the mind no less than in those of the body we can see the manifestation of the healing power of nature so familiar to the physician. Nature itself in ways far beyond our comprehension is constantly seeking to heal and to save. All that the best physician can do is to help nature in removing the obstacles to the free flow of life-giving forces. Nor does nature wait for the physician to act. This is perhaps even more true in the mental realm than it is in the physical. Man's power to help is very limited and nature itself is the chief actor in most of the cures that are actually effected. The acute disorders thus represent nature's attempts to get rid of the malignant sets and attitudes that are blocking development. They may also be looked upon as the resolution of the character elements present in the personality, analogous perhaps to the precipitation of the chemicals in a solution when a catalyzer is added. To predict the outcome in any particular case, once the physical factors have been evaluated, the best means is to take stock of the moral factors involved. This is of course no simple matter. The problem is a spiritual one in the strict sense of that term. We must look back of the outward symptoms to the inner meaning of the experience in terms of the patient's own picture of himself and of his own scale of values. What do the symptoms mean as regards the inner forces and motivations which make either for life or for death, for renewal or for destruction? These are the questions we must be able to answer if we are going to be able to recognize those cases which will repay intensive treatment and those that will not. In spite of the complexity of the problem and the elusiveness of the factors involved, we may on the basis of this study set down certain objective indications which will assist us in arriving at the inner meaning of a particular experience and thus forming an intelligent opinion regarding the direction in which the patient is likely to go.

1. The chances of recovery depend in large measure upon the possibility of making an adjustment in the life situation which will be acceptable to the patient. Where the situation is lacking in constructive factors and admits of no solution, where the patient has nothing to come back to, he may indeed be restored temporarily but he is not likely to remain well. Where, on the other hand, the outlook is hopeful, where the patient has ability, where he is acceptable to his social group and where the instinctual claims are not too completely in control, there the outlook for recovery is good.

2. The significance of reaction patterns must be carefully weighed. A sharp distinction must be drawn between those which represent the end results of malignant character tendencies, and the acute disturbances with their characteristic ideas of death, of cosmic catastrophe and cosmic identification. The latter, as we have seen, are to be regarded as attempts to break up the sets and attitudes which stand in the way of normal growth and function-

ing and to make possible a reorganization. The more sudden the
onset and the more acute the disturbance, the more likely the
patient is to recover, provided he can be protected from self-injury
and from physical infection and exhaustion. In many cases the
acute disturbance serves to change a malignant formation into a
benign reaction. The acute disturbances tend either to make or
to break. They may send the patient to the back wards, there to
remain as a hopeless wreck, or they may send him back into the
community in better shape than he had been for years. The outcome will depend upon the elements which are present, particularly upon the presence or absence of an acceptable nucleus of
purpose around which the new self can be formed.

3. Suffering may be looked upon as remedial. So long as the
patient is suffering and has a true appreciation of the seriousness
of the ordeal through which he is passing, there is ground for hope
that his condition may improve. The presence of inappropriate
moods and attitudes is a bad sign. Facetiousness of the manic
variety is perhaps an exception, though it may indicate that the
sufferer is not likely to achieve an enduring solution of his problem. But the significance of easy pleasure-taking during the
stormy phases of schizophrenia, particularly that of the erotic variety, is accurately represented by the old Greek legend of Proser-
pina and the pomegranate seeds. The sufferer remains in Hades.
Equally ominous are surly and bitter attitudes.

4. Attitudes of frankness and self-blame are favorable indications. Unless there are complicating factors those who commit
" the unpardonable sin " are likely to get well. So also do most
of those who are able to bring themselves to talk over their real
problems with someone who understands. If that can be brought
about the suffering and the danger of a severe upheaval may be
avoided.

5. " Voices " and other hallucinations indicate a stirring of the
deeper levels of the mental life, something which in itself may be
helpful as well as destructive. Their chief significance lies in what
they may reveal as to the inner trends and attitudes. What the

voices say is always the important question, not the mere fact of hearing voices.

6. Great caution must be exercised in passing judgment on the basis of objective behavior alone. What we need to know is the meaning of the particular behavior to the patient and its relationship to his accepted objectives. Two patients may do something equally disgusting. One does it under the compulsion of some need for self-punishment; the other as an expression of his baser nature. It is obvious that from the standpoint of prognosis the significance of such behavior is vastly different in the two cases.

The fact that in the acute disturbances of the problem-solving variety religious concern is so generally present suggests that we are hardly in position to form an intelligent judgment regarding the meaning of these experiences until after we have made a study of religious experience at its best and have considered the significance of the frequent association of the mystical and the pathological. This I shall attempt to do in the next chapter.

II

SOME SUCCESSFUL EXPLORERS

ACCORDING TO THE Book of Acts, Paul's account of his strange experience on the road to Damascus was received by the Roman governor with the comment, " Paul, thou art beside thyself. Much learning doth make thee mad." That remark has a familiar ring. It places the label of insanity upon a case of religious experience and it offers a common alibi. Most of those who are brought to mental hospitals are said by their friends to have overstudied or overworked or else to have fallen on their heads when they were youngsters. That the Roman governor was ready with such an alibi indicates that he was well-disposed toward Paul. Nevertheless Paul's experience to him was madness.

All down through the ages the experiences of men of religious genius have been subjected to this same galling suspicion. Never has this been more true than in our present sophisticated age and among the experts in mental abnormalities. For any man to assert, as Paul did, that he has heard a voice from on high, is in itself presumptive evidence of a psychosis, in the minds of most psychiatrists. Our present-day experts might not accept the Roman governor's explanation, but they would probably agree with his diagnosis in case Paul should appear before them in some new incarnation and offer such a tale. And for such a judgment there is much justification. They can point to countless persons with definitely disordered minds who claim to have had just such experiences as Paul described. And in many of our religious geniuses and mystics we can hardly fail to recognize features that are definitely psychopathic.

Paul and the men of his time would not for a moment deny that there was a certain relationship between his experience and those of the insane. They explained them all in terms of possession. But they drew a distinction which our present-day experts do not usually draw. They recognized possession by good spirits as well as by evil spirits. They thus took account of the values involved. We notice that in the New Testament, instead of speaking of a man as insane, it is said he was possessed by a demon; the faith in Jesus was based on the view that he, by the Spirit of God, was able to cast out the demons. He also was possessed, but possessed by the Holy Spirit (Matt. 12:22–9). Herein also, to Paul, lay the great significance of what had happened on the road to Damascus. The spirit of the Lord had appeared to him and taken possession of him so that it was no longer he that lived but Christ that lived in him (Gal. 2:20).

If we had to choose between the ancient explanation of mental illness in terms of possession, taking account of the character of the possessing spirits, and the modern mechanistic explanation which regards all abnormal experiences alike as psychopathic and calling for segregation, I for one would prefer the ancient explanation as truer to the facts and preferable from the standpoint of social welfare. Fortunately we are not limited to such an alternative. We are however faced with a definite challenge to find an explanation which shall be in accord with the wider range of facts revealed by modern science and shall take account of the constructive experiences of the man of genius as well as of the destructive experiences of the psychotic. That challenge we are ready to accept.

The study which we have just made of the experiences of mental patients has furnished us with a working hypothesis with which we may now approach the experiences of our men of religious genius. According to that hypothesis certain types of mental disorder are not in themselves evils but problem-solving experiences. They are attempts at reorganization in which the entire personality, to its bottommost depths, is aroused and its forces marshaled to meet the danger of personal failure and isolation. According to this hypothesis the primary evil in functional disorders lies in the realm of personal relationship, particularly to that which is for most men represented by the idea of God. The psychotic individual is characteristically one who, accepting the standards and ideals implanted by his early guides, has found within himself such marked deviation that he has been unable to face the inner bar of judgment except at the cost of severe emotional disturbance. In the more malignant types the sufferer has made no attempts to do so. He has either drifted along unresistingly, or else he has distorted his beliefs in order to maintain his sense of security. The acute disturbances, on the other hand, arise out of awareness of danger. The sufferer is facing what for him are the great and abiding issues of life and death and of his own relationship to the universe. He thus shows invariably marked religious concern. Such disturbances, as we have seen, tend either to make or break. Even those whose beliefs have been warped in the effort to interpret some unhappy life situation in terms favorable to their self-respect may, through the disturbance, find release and emerge into new life and hope. The emotional disturbance thus serves to break up malignant sets and attitudes and to make possible a new synthesis.

We may therefore begin the study of cases of recognized religious experience with the assumption that, even in definitely psychotic cases, emotional disturbances may be purposive and constructive. They may, and sometimes do, succeed in setting an individual free from what has been blocking his development, and in effecting a reorganization of the personality.

Material for such a study is not lacking. The Christian church has long recognized the significance of the inner conflict, and the classical description of such conflicts is that which Paul of Tarsus gives us in the seventh chapter of Romans:

I find then the law that to me who would do good evil is present. For I delight in the law of God after the inward man: but I see a different law in my members warring against the law of my mind and bringing me into captivity under the law of sin which is in my members. Wretched man that I am! who shall deliver me out of the body of this death?

Now Paul did not stop with his graphic description of the inner conflict. He believed that he had found the way out, and his experience and his teaching have set the pattern for the activities of the Christian church in its attempt to help the sick of soul. During all the centuries which have intervened since he enunciated his doctrine of the thralldom to the flesh and release through the spirit, the church has been seeking to save souls by the process of conversion and its records abound with accounts of spontaneous happy solutions of just such life situations as we have seen in the case of Albert W. But although such conversion experiences have been far from rare, the material available for our purpose is definitely limited. What we want is authentic records of experiences comparable in severity to those which we see in the hospital, but experiences in which the outcome has unquestioned validity from the standpoint of the results attained.[1] Such cases are not so common. Not many such persons find their way into or out of our mental hospitals where their histories are subjected to detached and comprehensive scrutiny. As to biographies and autobiographies, these are apt to be silent on those sections of their experience with which this study is concerned. This is particularly likely to be true of the sophisticated men of today, who are not unaware of the psychiatrist's attitude toward " voices " and who have a natural disinclination for casting their pearls before unsympathetic eyes. We must therefore turn back to the time of a faith more naïve for some of our best sources. Among these there is none more illuminating, from the standpoint of inquiry, than the autobiography of George Fox, the great founder of the Society of Friends.

George Fox has left us a remarkable account of his religious experience in a document known as his *Journal*.[2] The title is somewhat misleading, for the book is really a story of his life written chiefly during his imprisonment in Worcester Jail when he was

---

[1] I am assuming that for our inquiry the important contrast is not between what is normal and what is pathological in religious experience, but between victory and defeat on the battlefield of the inner life.

[2] Available in several editions. Our references are to the somewhat abridged edition edited by Rufus M. Jones under the title of *George Fox: An Autobiography* (Philadelphia, Ferris and Leach, 1903).

about fifty years old. But even though the account of the experience in which we are particularly interested is colored by his later experiences and attitudes, that account is unquestionably authentic and to the highest degree self-revealing.

What strikes us first of all as we read Fox's *Journal* in the light of the facts we have just been considering, is the severity of the experience through which he passed in his early twenties. We find in him the entire constellation of ideas which we have seen to be characteristic of those acute upheavals of the personality to which generally we give the name of " catatonic dementia praecox." Many of these ideas he carried with him throughout his entire active ministry. He considered himself the unique spokesman of the Lord to the people of his own generation, comparable only to the old Hebrew prophets. Passage after passage shows cosmic identification in its most unmistakable form (cf. pp. 120, 140, 149, 166). Repeatedly also he proclaimed " the day of the Lord that was coming upon all flesh " (pp. 102, 130, 141, 149, 150). He felt that he had been brought through the very ocean of darkness and death and through and over the power of Satan, even through that darkness which covered all the world and which chained down all and shut up all in death (p. 89). He felt that he had experienced the new birth (p. 102). His eyes were opened so that he saw that which was without end, things that cannot be uttered (p. 88). The whole creation was opened to him (p. 97). He was thus the recipient of direct revelations from God and he never acted on any important or even unimportant matter except in obedience to an " opening." Here then are all those ideas which we have seen in Albert W. and have found to be characteristic of the acute disturbance. The presumption which this fact establishes finds ample confirmation in what Fox tells us of the disturbed period which began in his nineteenth year and continued until his twenty-third. With the beginning of this disturbance he left his relations and broke off all familiarity or fellowship with young or old (p. 68). Strong temptations to despair came upon him (p. 69). He fasted much, walked abroad in solitary places, and often took his Bible and sat in hollow trees and lonesome places until night came on and frequently in the night walked mournfully about by himself (p. 79). The tempter charged him with having sinned against the Holy Ghost. It was impossible to declare the misery he was in, so great and heavy it was (p. 89). From the account that he gives it seems clear that if Fox were living today and were sent during such a disturbed period to a mental hospital, there would be scarcely any disagreement on the part of the staff as to his need of hospitalization or as to the label to be attached to the case.

But we are also struck by the power, the courage, the depth and tenderness of feeling, the clear insight and intelligence and the remarkable influence over men which his story reveals. Wherever he went he won followers. Even the Great Protector was moved to tears at his words (pp. 213–15), and at the time of his death he was the leader of a group of some forty thousand devoted followers. He seems to have grown in the directions of inner unification and social outreach and effectiveness. Certainly the history of the Society of Friends bears witness to the wholesome influence of his life and teachings. In the light of his own history and of that of his followers, we may raise the question whether he may not have been right in believing himself comparable to the old Hebrew prophets. We thus find ourselves confronted with the problem of the origin and significance of the religious insights of the human race, and we find support for the view that the experiences of Albert W. and of his fellow sufferers, painful and unsatisfactory though they may be, may indeed throw some light upon this important and baffling problem.

Our first task will be to determine what there was in the character of George Fox which may explain the difference in outcome between his case and that of Albert W. We may begin by asking, What were the forces or tendencies involved in the disturbance which led Fox into his prophetic career?

According to Fox's story the disturbance grew out of an incident which to us seems rather trivial. He was invited by a cousin and a friend to share part of a jug of beer with them. The invitation he accepted promptly. When they had drunk a glass apiece the two others proposed a drinking contest to be paid for by the one who quit first. Fox immediately departed and that night he could not sleep, but walked up and down, praying in great distress until finally he received the charge, " Thou seest how young people go together into vanity and old people into the earth; thou must forsake all, young and old, keep out of all, and be as a stranger unto all " (*Journal,* p. 68). What was there in this beer-drinking incident to produce the three to four years of profound disturbance that followed?

The facts considered in our hospital cases have shown us that we are not to look for the explanation of such disturbances in the immediate occasion which precipitates them. Most acute disturbances and upheavals come as the result of an accumulation of strains and stresses. The break occurs when the load becomes too heavy, and the occasion which precipitates it is usually a mere last straw.[3] To explain the disturbance we must therefore examine the previous history. In Fox's case certain facts are clear. While he tells us only a little concerning his early years, what he does tell is significant. He reveals himself as an extremely serious-minded boy who accepted unquestioningly the teachings of his early guides, one who took his religion very seriously and who seems to have been singularly free from the grosser sex maladjustments, which figure so prominently in most of our hospital cases. At least, he is able to say, as he looks back upon his boyhood, that he knew purity and righteousness and that he acted faithfully in all things, both inwardly to God and outwardly to man (p. 66).

In view of Fox's unflinching honesty and of the type of solution actually achieved, there seems to be no reason to doubt that statement. It is moreover clear that his sense of humor was deficient, that he was extremely sensitive and extremely stubborn, that he associated very little with other boys and that he was laughed at by them and by other " rude persons." Even though, as he says, he would leave them alone and go his way, he must certainly have felt his isolation very keenly (*Journal,* p. 67). The point of the beer-drinking incident would then lie in the fact that his cousin and his

[3] See preceding chapter, pp. 30–31.

friend were having some fun at his expense, and even though they were professing Christians, in proposing a drinking bout they had allied themselves with the hoodlum element who made life so miserable for him. We may furthermore assume that Fox had made a virtue of his isolation and had sought to maintain his self-respect by an attitude of righteous horror over the excesses of other young men of his age. In any case, the incident served as the last straw, and with it came the prolonged and severe disturbance.

We may notice that this disturbance began in the way which we have found to be characteristic of our acutely disturbed hospital cases. He had an experience which he interpreted as supernatural in origin. The Lord spoke to him. The message did not condemn him. It merely exiled him from his fellows (*ibid.*, p. 68). It was thus a recognition and also an acceptance of the fact of his isolation. It was even implicitly a commission. In any case it was an experience so tremendous that it destroyed the structure upon which his judgments had been based and compelled a revaluation of values. He was thus thrown into a protracted period of confusion and distress.

From this disturbance he began to emerge with the " opening " that training at Oxford or Cambridge was not enough to " fit and qualify men to be ministers of Christ " (*ibid.* p. 75). He states that this struck at Priest Stephen's ministry. It is probable that it did something far more important than that. It seems to have opened a new path for himself and to have given him a new goal in life. Other openings followed which enabled him to rebuild his life and to work out his *Weltanschauung*. In this there is nothing unusual. It is merely an exemplification of the principle that there can be no mental functioning without a body of assumptions in regard to ourselves and the universe which serves as the foundation of our reasoning processes. And just as the disorder itself is a result of the upsetting of these assumptions, so recovery comes with their reorganization. In our hospital cases we have found three types of solutions: the individual may remain at the chaotic level; he may resume his previous body of beliefs and assumptions; or he may rebuild his shattered faith in himself on the basis of some new idea or ideas which have come with the disturbance. In the latter case, the ideas which serve as the basis of reconstruction are usually of the sort that others cannot accept, but they do in some measure enable him to keep his head above water and to go on functioning as a self-respecting unit. Over and over again, in our hospital cases, we see something resembling order emerging from the chaos as soon as this process of systematization takes place. Among such reconstructions there are two common types: those in which faith in one's self is maintained by a transfer of blame, and those in which faith is maintained by delusions of self-importance. Fox bears a close relationship to the latter group. But he also presents a sharp contrast to the common grandiose paranoic. By virtue of the simple honesty and fidelity and earnestness of purpose which had characterized him from childhood, he succeeded in finding his way through the wilderness to a commanding point of view which enabled him to bring order and even something of beauty out of the chaos through which he had passed. His experience had served to open up to him the inner world throughout its entire range, and he emerged from that disturbance to live upon a new and higher level. His life was rebuilt stronger and more beautiful than it had been before.[4] This new structure was built upon ideas and insights which had come to him through the disturbance. Some of them may seem to us delusional misinterpretations. But there are also insights of great social value. He became the bearer of a message to which the people of his time were ready to listen, and with the increasing social support which thus came to him, his own eccentricities became less marked.

Not only did Fox carry with him from out of the disturbed period certain ideas and insights which continued to dominate his life, but he also continued throughout his career to trust his "openings." Never did he act in any matter, even though of minor importance, except in obedience to an opening. The

---

[4] Freud, *Psychoanalytische Bemerkungen ueber einen autobiographisch beschriebenen Fall von Paranoia* (Neurosenlehre: Dritte Folge. Leipzig, Franz Deuticke, 1921), p. 259.

lengths to which he went in obeying these openings may be seen in his strange account of his visit to Lichfield. We see him here, in obedience to the command of the Lord, taking off his shoes in midwinter and walking up and down the streets on a market day, crying out, " Woe to the bloody city of Lichfield." It is true that this incident occurred shortly after his release from a long and severe imprisonment, a fact which may account for his extremely bizarre behavior, but it is to be noted that the account is written at least fifteen years later and yet it does not occur to him to question the validity of the prompting. He does indeed express surprise that no one laid hands upon him. He also wonders why he should have been called upon to denounce Lichfield as " bloody," for he recognizes that no more blood seems to have been spilt in Lichfield than in the neighboring towns, but he arrives finally at the remarkable explanation that in Emperor Diocletian's time a thousand Christians were martyred in Lichfield (pp. 132-3).

The surprising thing is that any man who obeyed his hunches so implicitly as Fox did should not have got into more serious difficulties. Instead of that, however, the openings seem to have become more and more trustworthy. In explanation three contributing factors may be suggested: In the first place, he is constantly on his guard against the lure of his own wishes and obeys the openings implicitly only when they run counter to his wishes. We thus notice that whenever Fox hears of a situation which is difficult or dangerous, he usually gets an opening which sends him into it.[5] Where his wishes are involved, we see him, as at the time of his marriage, carefully checking up his openings by the judgment and advice of his friends (pp. 468-9). We may also be sure that with the passage of time he came to exercise his critical judgment far more than he was aware. The third factor would be the steady development in the direction of discipline and unification of character. The openings would thus tend to become more and more dependable, just as the automatic responses of the skilled baseball player or proficient pianist, as compared with the clumsy movements of the beginner.

[5] Cf., pp. 181, 277, 290, 311, 392, 405.

It is of great interest to note that although as a young man Fox passed through four years of profound mental disorder, there was no further difficulty until twenty years later, and then only as the result of a special situation. In the course of his arduous ministry he spent many years in prison, often in solitary confinement and under the most trying conditions. For sheer horror it is difficult to match his account of the conditions of his imprisonment in Doomsdale in Launceston Dungeon (p. 256). But all this he endured with remarkable fortitude and unshaken faith in himself and in his cause. But when in his forty-fifth year his followers were undergoing a fierce persecution and he himself was unmolested, he went through a second severe disturbance. At this time, he tells us, he was under great sorrows and oppressions, warring in spirit against the evil spirits that warred against truth and friends. He was brought into the deep and saw all the religions of the world and the people that lived in them. He was at this time so sick that few thought he could live, but when the fury of the persecutions abated he recovered (pp. 476–81).

This analysis of Fox's religious experience indicates that it was truly comparable to that of Albert W. and his fellow sufferers of the acutely disturbed type. Fox showed the entire constellation of ideas which we have seen in Albert and have found to be characteristic of acute disturbances generally. There seems to be no question as to his having passed through an acute emotional upheaval. But there are also some differences. In contrast to the great body of acute cases in our research group, for whom the disturbance represented an awareness of danger which in many cases was already an accomplished fact before the victim awoke to it, he shares with Albert W. the earnest striving after the better life as a volitional nucleus around which a reorganization might take place. With Albert he stands sharply contrasted in the essential integrity of character which he brought to the disturbed period. Albert was a composite of conflicting elements which could not go on forever side by side but had to fight it out for the mastery. Fox, on the other hand, came to the disturbed period conscious of his " innocency and honesty." With him the difficulty seems to have been that his extreme earnestness of purpose, together with his utter lack of any sense of humor, had made him an object of ridicule. This fact may explain the great contrast in the type of solution arrived at as compared with the hospital cases.

The hospital cases showed nothing better than a clearing up of certain malignant tendencies and a return to previously " normal " views and attitudes, while a large proportion of them remained on the level of disorganization, and still others have made a reconstruction on a delusional basis. Fox, on the other hand, emerged from the disturbance with certain socially valuable insights and a new purpose in life. He was thus able to assimilate the entire experience through which he had passed and to bring to men of his generation a message in regard to those ultimate realities with which in his disturbance he had been faced. The result in his case was progressive unification on a plane conceived of as universal.

Another case of great interest from our point of view is that of George Fox's contemporary, John Bunyan. Bunyan has left us a graphic account of a four-year period of disturbance through which he passed in his early twenties. As in the case of Fox, and also of the hospital cases, this disturbance began with an experience which he interpreted as a manifestation of the supernatural. It was characterized by alternating moods of elation and depression, of hope and despair, hyper-suggestibility, morbid conscientiousness, and the obsessive fear that he had committed the unpardonable sin. The inner conflict was dramatized in the form of a contest between two sets of scripture texts which kept darting into his mind — one set condemnatory, reminding him of Esau and the sale of his birthright; the other set comforting, giving assurance of forgiveness. The solution came with the conviction that " the word of grace " was stronger than that of Esau.

Like Fox, Bunyan, even in his mature years, never questioned the supernatural origin of these obsessive texts. He merely attributed one set to the devil and lost his fear of them through his faith in the power and mercy of the Lord. It is furthermore to be noted that in later years he derived much comfort and help from the scriptural texts which continued still to dart into his mind, a striking illustration of the principle that meaning, and not mechanism, is the significant thing in mental illness.

Bunyan's disturbance was apparently of a somewhat different type than that of Fox. The regression was not so profound. At least there is no evidence that he had the set of ideas which we have found to be characteristic of the deeper disturbances. We need therefore only consider his experience briefly as an example of unquestionable mental disorder which was at the same time, no less unquestionably, religious experience of the problem-solving type. The pathological features in his experience have been set forth very clearly by Professor Josiah Royce of Harvard University in his interesting study of " The Case of John Bunyan," which he wrote toward the end of the last century. Professor Royce arrives at the conclusion that " Bunyan was a man of genius who bore with a heroic perseverance a heavy and morbid load of nervous ill and in the end won a mastery over it." [6] Bunyan himself was of another opinion. His account of his experience bears the title, " Grace Abounding to the Chief of Sinners." In the subtitle we learn that this was written " for the Support of the Weak and Tempted People of God." Clearly he looked upon it as constructive religious experience. Such a view is quite in line with our findings and this case gives striking support to our hypothesis. Certainly Bunyan, like Fox, emerged from the disturbed period with a mind sensitized to the realities of the inner world. Instead therefore of being a man of genius *in spite of* his " heavy and morbid load of nervous ill," we may in the light of this study venture the conclusion that he was a man of genius precisely *because of* that experience and of its triumphant outcome. Through that experience this more or less commonplace village tinker was launched upon the adventurous journey which he has described so vividly in his *Pilgrim's Progress*. Through it he was given a new vision and a new purpose in life which made him a respected leader among men of his time. This happy outcome may be explained in his case, as also in the case of Fox, by the fact that he

[6] *Studies in Good and Evil* (New York, D. Appleton, 1898), p. 30.

had for some time been an earnest seeker after the better life and he brought to the disturbed period a well-developed set of interests and purposes which served as the organizing center of his new philosophy of life.

More nearly similar to the case of George Fox as regards the type of disturbance is the case of Emmanuel Swedenborg. While Swedenborg has given us no autobiography, he has left us a most revealing " Spiritual Diary," which contains a careful record of his dreams during the period of acute conflict. This [7] together with his voluminous writings gives us a fairly clear picture of the man and of the profound upheaval through which he passed in the middle of his sixth decade. At the time this disturbance came on, Swedenborg, a man of influential family and independent means, was probably the outstanding Swedish scholar of the early eighteenth century. He was a man of colossal learning, a veritable encyclopedia of the human knowledge of that time. His sex adjustments were, however, unsatisfactory. He was unmarried, and the record of his dreams indicates clearly a deep sense of unworthiness as a primary factor in the disturbance. Here again we find at the outset of the disturbed period an experience interpreted as a manifestation of the superpersonal. According to his own statement, the Lord himself appeared to him and opened his sight into the spiritual world and enabled him to converse with spirits.[8] From this disturbance he emerged with a new set of interests and a new philosophy of life. The remainder of his life was marked by tremendous productivity and increasing influence. Central in his teaching was the idea of the imminent second advent of the Lord, and of the New Jerusalem coming down from heaven upon earth. It is likewise clear that he regarded himself as especially commissioned of the Lord to reveal the secrets of the spiritual world to the people of his time. Although Emerson has given to Swedenborg a place among the great heroes of all time, and although he left behind him a significant group of followers — the

---

[7] Tafel, *Documents Concerning Swedenborg* (London, Swedenborg Society, 1875), vol. 2, pt. 1, documents 208–9.

[8] *Ibid.*, vol. 1, document 2, pp. 7–8.

group which produced William James and implanted the interests which appear in his *Varieties of Religious Experience* — I find it difficult to place him in the same rank with Fox and Bunyan. His chief interests seem to have been in the occult rather than in the ethical. He wrote on such subjects as "Heaven and Hell," "Spiritual Marriage," and the like. His influence, moreover, seems to have been based very largely upon his clairvoyant faculties.

Among the old Hebrew prophets with whom Fox compared himself, the case of Ezekiel is of peculiar interest from the standpoint of this study. The Book of Ezekiel begins with the statement that the heavens were opened and Ezekiel saw visions of God, that the word of Jehovah came expressly unto him and the hand of Jehovah was laid upon him. It goes on to describe certain of these visions, which are full of all sorts of archaic symbolism of the kind which we find so characteristically among our acutely disturbed patients. Then comes his commission to preach to the House of Israel a message of wrath and doom. Ezekiel himself was to be the living embodiment and symbol of the rebellious nation. He was to act out all that was to befall them. He was thus required to lie 340 days upon his left side in order to represent the years of their punishment. He was required to lie forty days upon his right side to represent forty years of siege. He was moreover required, though later released from the command, to bake barley cakes compounded with human dung, and to do this in the sight of all, in order to set forth the message that the people of Israel were to eat their bread unclean in the sight of the nations (chap. 4). Throughout, Ezekiel is the mouthpiece of Jehovah (3:4), Jehovah's hand is heavy upon him (3:14). Jehovah opens his mouth (3:22; 33:22), Jehovah makes him dumb (3:26; 33:22). The spirit lifts him up between heaven and earth (8:3). Other instances might be cited but these may suffice to show in the case of Ezekiel the characteristic ideas of cosmic catastrophe, cosmic identification and mission, the archaic symbolism, and the authority of experiences interpreted as possession, which we encounter over and over again in our acutely disturbed patients. But along with these abnormal manifestations we find, as we found also in Fox and Bunyan, the integrity of character and sincerity of purpose which enabled him to emerge on a higher level with a fine moral insight and increasing practical judgment as a true spokesman for that which was forward-looking and best in the spirit of his people.

Jeremiah is likewise very interesting from the standpoint of our inquiry. In him also we see the same set of ideas which we found to be characteristic of the acute upheavals and which we have seen also in Fox and Swedenborg and Ezekiel. Jeremiah feels himself the bearer of a message concerning the fate of his people. This message is at first one of doom. He even carries it to the point of insisting that King Zedekiah must surrender his people to the Babylonians, a position which, not surprisingly, subjects him to the charge of treason on the part of the Hebrew warriors. After Jerusalem's fall, his message becomes one of hope and encouragement. For his prophetic task he feels himself especially chosen of the Lord, even before he was born (1:5). The Lord puts his words into his mouth and sets him over nations and over kingdoms to root out and to pull down and to destroy, to build and to plant (1:9, 10). The Lord makes him a brazen wall against which the people could not prevail. He feels himself merely a passive instrument in the hands of the Lord. The word of the Lord is in his heart as a burning fire so that he cannot stay it. The Lord is too strong for him. He speaks just what the Lord puts into his mouth, and he complains bitterly because the word he had spoken in the name of the Lord has not come true and he has thus become an object of derision to his enemies. He reproaches the Lord with having deceived him and he curses the day wherein he had been born (chap. 20). He thus takes us into his confidence and permits us to see something of his misgivings and conflicts in the carrying out of his prophetic task. Very striking is the answer of the Lord to his complainings: " If thou becomest again mine, thou mayest again be my servant, and if thou freest thy better self from the vile, then shalt thou be as my mouth " (15:9). The identification with the Lord is however almost constant with him. So far, in fact, did he carry it as to look upon his own enemies and those who disagreed with him as enemies of the Lord and to expect the Lord to wreak vengeance upon them (15:15; 17:18).

In Jeremiah, as in Ezekiel, we find the tendency to see a message from the Lord in some object or happening which he might encounter. A branch of an almond tree is thus a symbol that the Lord will watch over his words to perform them. A boiling cauldron facing toward the north tells him that disaster is brewing for his people from the direction of the north. A vessel broken in the hands of the potter represents to him the plan of the Lord to break refractory Israel and then to make them again a new vessel. On one occasion he places a yoke about his neck to symbolize his message that his people were to be taken captive. In all this we may recognize the vision of the poet verging upon the tendency of the psychotic to read hidden meanings into what he sees about him.

We thus see that Jeremiah shares with certain types of patients, whom we can observe today in our hospitals, the tendency to accept implicitly the promptings which come into his mind as of supernatural origin and divine authority. He also occupies himself with a message of doom which is to come upon all his people and he identifies himself with Jehovah, their Lord, as his chosen servant and spokesman. In contrast with the ordinary patient, however, is the subject matter with which he is concerned and the results which he attains. He is preoccupied with the welfare of his people and he achieves a real grasp of the problems relating to it. Even though his message is one of doom, it is yet characterized by a marvelous depth and tenderness of feeling and by insights of rare penetration and beauty.

Similar characteristics are found in others of the Hebrew prophets. They proclaimed a coming day of doom and looked upon themselves as the spokesmen of Jehovah, speaking with an authoritative " Thus saith the Lord " which was for them something much more than a stereotyped phrase. We thus find in nearly all the Hebrew prophets clear indications of that constellation of ideas which suggests that they may in some measure have shared the experience of Fox, of Swedenborg, of Albert W., and of acute upheavals generally. There is however one striking characteristic of all these Hebrew prophets. Their central concern was not with the problem of personal salvation, but with that of their people. The question therefore arises whether some of them, like Fox, may not have so completely identified themselves with their people that they went down into the depths with their people in their sufferings.[9] Their severe disturbance might thus be explainable not so much in terms of their own personal conflicts and inner difficulties as in terms of group danger. They would thus be those who were fine enough and farseeing enough to feel with and for their nation and to lead that nation to a racial self-consciousness which served, not merely to carry them through the immediate crises, but which has persisted throughout the centuries in spite of their being scattered far and wide throughout the world. More than that, these men were able to arrive at an interpretation of the sufferings of their people which, in the depth of its insight and in the sureness of its moral understanding, remains among the finest expressions of the spirit of man.

Among the men who figure in biblical history, there is none concerning whom we have records so full and so authentic as Saul of Tarsus. Neither is there anyone whose experience is of greater importance for our inquiry. We know not merely from the Book of Acts, but from personal letters of his own, whose authenticity is scarcely questioned, that he went through a cataclysmic experience which resulted in the reorganization of his entire life. We also see in him the same constellation of ideas which were found in Fox, in Swedenborg, in Ezekiel, in Jeremiah, and in acutely disturbed hospital patients. He believed that the Lord had appeared to him by direct revelation, that this experience was similar to the resurrection appearances of Jesus to his disciples, and that this fact entitled him to an authority equal to that of the disciples of Jesus. He proclaimed the second coming of the Lord, and although this belief was already held by the early Christians, it was undoubtedly based primarily upon his own experience. He refers repeatedly to his having " died in Christ " (2 Cor. 4:11 ff.; Gal. 2:19–20; Phil. 3:10), and along with this, to

[9] I, p. 73.

his " being raised again with Christ " (Cor. 4:14) and to the
" Christ that lived in him " (Phil. 2:20, 4). We have thus not
merely ideas of death and of rebirth or renewal, but also, apparently, a constructive interpretation of the experience which
leads so many of our patients to identify themselves with Christ
or with God. He also records certain mystical experiences in
which he was caught up into the third heaven and heard unspeak-
able words which it is not lawful for man to utter (2 Cor. 12:2–4).
All through his ministry he believed himself guided and inspired
by the spirit of God. In Paul we have, moreover, a man of abounding vitality, of sound practical judgment and of fine moral judgment who, more than any others of the followers of Jesus, was
instrumental in making Christianity a world-wide religion.

In trying to understand the forces at work in this experience
on the road to Damascus, we may ask first of all why it was that
this aristocratic, well-educated, able young Jew should have been
so tremendously concerned about this obscure little sect of Christians.

Not many facts are given us regarding the early life of Paul,
but a few things are clear. He was a Jew of the Dispersion. He
was born and raised in Tarsus, a city in which Greek influence was
fairly strong. His family was well-to-do and influential, and he
had received the best education obtainable in that period and
region, apparently with the idea of becoming a rabbi. His first
appearance on the scene of New Testament history is as a furious
persecutor of the Christians. He had a leading part in the stoning
of Stephen and at the very moment of his conversion was on his
way to Damascus for the purpose of putting certain unhappy
Christians into prison.

In trying to understand the forces at work in this experience
on the road to Damascus, we may ask first of all why it was that
this aristocratic, well-educated, able young Jew should have been
so tremendously concerned about this obscure little sect of Christians.

We may note, first of all, that Paul was a member of a minority group which was striving to maintain its racial integrity
against the onslaughts of a dominant surrounding culture. This
it sought to do by a loyalty to the past and a magnification of the
divisive race symbols. The study of any similar groups today —
and we can find plenty of them in our racial or foreign language
churches in America — reveals that there nearly always results

that tragedy of loyalty, the loss of perspective, and the tendency to overemphasize the petty and the trivial and the divisive.

But this consideration is not sufficient to account for bigotry and intolerance carried to the extreme of putting to death those who differ. Whenever we find intolerance so intense we are justified in suspecting some deeper-seated personal difficulty. We may perhaps assume that it originates in some inner discomfort. We may assume then that Paul had a sore spot and that in some way the Christians had touched him on the raw. We may, moreover, hazard a guess as to the nature of that sore spot. If we may take the seventh chapter of Romans as in any sense autobiographical, he was having a hard time keeping his instinctual drives, the " flesh " as he calls it, under control and he was making use of the devices so common in the racial religions for the maintenance of his accepted loyalties. He was trying to obey " every jot and tittle of the law." He was substituting minor for major virtues and minor for major loyalties. He was thus not merely born a Pharisee but he was employing the pharisaic pattern.

If this supposition is correct we can easily understand why the early Christians and their teachings might have made him un-comfortable. They had a good deal to say about inward as against outward righteousness and Jesus had been unsparing in his denunciation of the religious group to which Paul belonged. He accused them of straining at the gnat and swallowing the camel. He said they were particular about outward appearances precisely because they were uneasy about what was inside, and that their overemphasis on trivialities was due precisely to their neglect of the weightier matters of the law. More than that, the Christians did away with the old nationalistic hope. Instead of looking forward to a time when some conquering son of David should come and lead them to victory and domination over other peoples, they were talking about a reign of love that was to follow upon some sort of world catastrophe. These considerations may perhaps make clear why the Christians touched him on the raw. He therefore sought to exterminate them because they made him uncomfortable. Even the deep impression made upon his sen-

sitive mind by the death of the martyr Stephen would only increase his persecutory zeal because it increased the discomfort.
And the persecutory zeal continued with increasing intensity until
the solution finally came in the overwhelming experience on the
road to Damascus. This experience seems to have been definitely
hallucinatory in character. From the account which he gives in
the letters to the Galatians and to the Corinthians, it is clear that
he thought that the risen Lord had appeared to him. According
to the Acts' account he saw a light and heard a voice and, if we
may believe the account as given in the twenty-sixth chapter,
something by no means incredible, he received right there in a
blinding flash of insight the commission to preach a gospel of
forgiveness and redemption to the Gentiles. In any case, this
experience became for him the organizing center of a new plan
of life. But such reorganizations do not come full-blown. Judging from what we see in our hospital cases we should expect this
experience to be followed by a period of confusion and disorder.
That such a period of disturbance did follow may be inferred from
his own statement that this experience on the road to Damascus
was followed by a trip into Arabia, and that it was only after
three years that he established connections with the Christian
group and began his active ministry (Gal. 1:17).

We see thus in Paul a man with a severe inner conflict who has
recourse to certain unsatisfactory protective devices, seeking to
suppress a troublesome conscience, until the tension reaches the
breaking point and the solution comes with cataclysmic sudden-
ness. In this there is nothing in Paul's story which could not be
duplicated in any of our mental hospitals. What is distinctive
in the case of Paul, as also in the case of Fox and Bunyan and
Swedenborg and Ezekiel and Jeremiah, is the intense sincerity
and earnestness of the man and the character of the solution arrived at, as measured by the social value of his insights and objectives and the degree of achievement attained. We rate Paul
among the great religious geniuses of the world because what
happened on the road to Damascus changed Paul the legalist into
Paul the prophet of the spirit, because it changed Paul the super-

patriot into Paul the great Apostle to the Gentiles, and Paul the persecutor of Jesus and his followers into the zealous missionary who carried the Christian gospel throughout the Roman world.

These particular men have been chosen from among the religious geniuses of the world because in the course of their development they passed through periods of emotional disturbance and upheaval comparable in severity to the experience of our acutely disturbed patients. We are thus proceeding on the assumption that the correct contrast is not between the pathological and the normal in religious experience but between spiritual defeat and spiritual victory, and that the more severe disturbances serve to isolate and throw into clear relief certain of the significant variables. Even though we have not found a large number who satisfy our requirements in the matter of type and of documentation, they may yet serve to provide us with rewarding leads. These cases all exemplify the association of the mystical and the pathological so frequent in the history of religion, and the comparison of these experiences with those of our acutely disturbed hospital cases has provided us with a basis for some generalizations regarding the nature and function of religion and the meaning of the cataclysmic experiences, whether their outcome be constructive or otherwise. Some of these generalizations will be left for later consideration, but a few observations are in order at this point.

Common to all these experiences is the narrowing of attention with which the experience is initiated. The individual becomes wholly absorbed in a narrow circle of ideas. In most cases this is accompanied by the loss of sleep carried to the point where the boundaries are lost between sleeping and waking. In this condition a man is half awake when he ought to be asleep and half asleep when he ought to be awake. In any case there is preoccupation and absorption so intense that the individual lapses into an abnormal condition suggestive of auto-hypnosis or trance. The conscious self is plunged into the lower strata of the mental life and finds itself surrounded by elemental and archaic thought forms. The individual thus feels himself in a strange new world in which previous experience and accepted standards of value do not apply. In the hospital cases this condition is induced nearly always under the dominance of fear. The patient is face to face with the realities of death and life. He is in consequence overwhelmed with terror which may or may not change into the uncertain glow of cosmic identification.

In the cases of the men of religious genius whom we have considered, the initial fear stage may or may not have been present, but cosmic identification in the form of a sense of union with the Greater-than-self is characteristic. In them it becomes no longer intermittent and uncertain but the foundation of a successful reorganization and transformation of the personality. This experience of union with the divine is probably the matrix of all religion. While it is by no means confined to the abnormal or pathological experiences, the feeling can be induced through the trance state, and techniques for inducing this trance state are much in evidence. Where the trance conditions are entered into under the dominance of faith and confidence, the effects may be on the whole steadying and beneficial. The dominance of fear is thus one of the reasons why the acute disturbances we see in the hospital are apt to be so destructive.

Common also to the two groups is the dynamic and purposive character of the experiences undergone. They seem to be attempts to solve problems, and those problems have to do with the personal destiny and with ultimate loyalties and values as seen through the eyes of the individual. Who am I? Why am I in this world? What's the matter? What is going to happen to me and to my friends? How can I save the situation? How can I make atonement for my mistakes and sins? How can I bring about a realization of the possibilities that ought to be? These are generally the questions in the focus of attention both in hospital experiences and in those of the men of religious genius. Probably those questions are central in any philosophy of life. Commonly the personal drama is projected upon a cosmic scale but its meaning remains the same. The tremendous impact of the experience is due to the sudden widening of the horizon and the sense of immediacy which is involved. Philosophy and theology are no longer theoretical and abstract problems. They are matters of life and death. Even though in many of the hospital cases the results are destructive, the disturbance itself is none the less constructive in purpose. It is better to die trying than not to try at all, better to run the risk of a dangerous operation than to drift unresistingly down to destruction.

In the men of religious genius whom we have studied, we have individuals of high potentiality who have been made over from more or less ordinary types into persons of enduring significance in the history of the world. This does not mean that experiences of the cataclysmic variety are to be sought after. The essential thing is that the individual should grow into his full stature. Steady and unbroken development is ever the ideal, but that ideal is not always possible. Wherever difficulties have been allowed to accumulate, there an emotional disturbance may be unavoidable if the true objectives are to be achieved. There is also the definite possibility that in some of our men of religious genius a stage of disturbance may represent the attainment of some new level of development and the coming of some new insight which compels a radical reorganization of the philosophy of life.

Our consideration of the cases of our successful explorers has served to reinforce the conclusion arrived at in our study of the less successful. The cataclysmic experiences, regardless of outcome, are manifestations of the power not ourselves that makes for health. They are nature's attempts to get rid of sets and attitudes that block growth, and to effect a reorganization of the personality. The outcome in any particular case is thus determined by the character elements present, particularly by the strength of the moral strivings and aspirations and the determined outreach after the unattained possibilities. Common to all our men of religious genius has been the presence of a will to righteousness and moral achievement. Even though faulty and imperfect, they had been struggling vigorously for the better life. The period of disturbance for them has represented the attempt of the better self to gain control, and because that better self was already well developed, the disturbance was as the casting off of an old skin by a molting reptile or the breaking of an eggshell by the chicken ready to be hatched. In any case, the cataclysmic experience was merely incidental to growth and development.

The association of the mystical and the pathological, which we have found both in the hospital cases and in the experiences of Fox and Bunyan and the rest, is now not difficult to understand. The explanation is to be found in the principle that religious concern and religious consciousness tend to appear wherever men are facing the issues of life and are seeking to become better.[10] Wherever this involves severe conflict pathological features are likely also to appear. In some cases the charge of pathology as applied to religious experience is due simply to the failure to recognize that such phenomena as hallucinations spring from the tapping of the deeper levels of the mental life, and that as such they are not necessarily symptomatic of mental disorder but may be creative and constructive. But in a large number of cases the association of the mystical and the pathological is due to the fact that a fundamental reorientation is a necessary stage in the development of the individual. Albert W. is thus in his disturbed period no more disorganized and scarcely less concerned about the spiritual world than was George Fox in his early twenties. In the archaic symbolism to which both gave expression there are striking similarities. But Fox, together with others of the great mystics, succeeded in doing something which Albert W. did not do. He succeeded in making certain insights which came to him in the disturbed period the organizing center of a socially valuable new self. He carried with him from out of the disturbance a continued outreach after the best and a continued fidelity to the promptings of his deeper self which enabled him to grow steadily in the direction of inner unification on a basis conceived of as universal.

[10] Dewey, *Reconstruction in Philosophy* (New York, Henry Holt and Co., 1920), p. 176.

III

GEORGE FOX AMONG THE DOCTORS

THE SURVEY OF the inner world which we have just completed has revealed the fact that there exists a close association between religious experience and the pathological. Not only do acutely disturbed mental patients show characteristically a keen awareness of the realm of unattained possibilities which, according to Professor Wieman, is the mark of the religious,[1] but they also in many cases interpret their experience in terms of mystical identification. On the other hand, we have found not a few men of outstanding religious genius who have passed through periods of acute mental disorder in the process of finding themselves. It becomes therefore a matter of no little importance to discover just what we have to offer to a man of the latter type today. Would George Fox in some present-day incarnation be any more likely to find those who understood the significance of his tremendous religious drive in its setting of pathological manifestations than was the case two hundred and eighty years ago?

We have seen how Fox, at the time of the first workings of the Lord in him when he was beset with great temptations to despair, went the rounds of the priests and ministers of the land seeking one who could speak to his condition; but no such man could he find. Let us now go with Fox and his problem to those who are accounted experts in this age of enlightenment, in order to discover how far we have advanced in the insights which will enable us to further and not to destroy the possibilities which in that dis-

[1] *The Wrestle of Religion with Truth* (New York, Macmillan Co., 1927), p. 135.

turbance were seeking to come to birth. Our analysis of Fox's experience has shown that he was, in his early twenties, in a condition of such disorder that if he were living today the question would at once arise, What shall we do with him? For the purpose of our inquiry it may be worth while to bring him before the doctors and have him examined. This procedure will have the double advantage of furnishing us an opportunity to examine the doctors as well as Fox. We may thus be able to determine what progress they have made toward the understanding of the religious concern which characterizes the acute disturbances which we find in our mental hospitals, and of the psychopathic manifestations which so frequently appear at some stage in the development of other men of religious genius besides Fox as well as in many others who are religious without attaining to the ranks of genius. This plan will furthermore enable me to make clear my indebtedness to those who have contributed most to my own thinking.

THE DOCTORS OF DIVINITY

Our first visit will be to a doctor of divinity. This, as we have seen, was Fox's own thought. It was to the priest and the minister of religion that he looked for help. We must not fail to recognize that we are giving them a very knotty problem, for Fox was as clearly psychotic as he was religious. He would hardly be ready to accept help or guidance. Our question will then concern itself with the attitude of present-day ministers of religion toward the sick of soul and the degree of understanding with which they approach it.

Ministers of religion can be found without difficulty in any part of the United States. Exclusive of Catholics and Negroes there are, according to the census report, some 135,000 ministers of religion in the United States; few families, even in the isolated country districts, are not within easy reach of some organized religious work. A survey of these ministers and of the groups to which they belong reveals a bewildering array of denominations and doctrines. Among these, three main groups may be distinguished which we may designate the evangelistic, the ecclesiastical and the liberal. Of these three groups the first is still the largest, even though its influence is steadily decreasing. According to the law of probabilities it is therefore a representative of this group that our patient will be likely to visit first.

1. The Evangelistic Group. Within the evangelistic group we find many and diverse tendencies, from the wild and primitive " Holy Roller " cults and the vagaries of the Pre-millenarian, to the staid correctness of the educated Calvinist. There is, however, one characteristic which is common to all. Their message derives its authority from tradition and concerns itself with the problem of salvation or rescue. Man's nature is regarded as innately bad and a " new birth " is necessary to salvation. This salvation, while not without a strong ethical content, is thought of largely in other-worldly terms. God is looked upon as a personal spirit who intervenes in human affairs. While many members of this group, at least among the older generation, are highly educated men, there is a general hostility to the results of modern scientific investigation, especially to the theory of evolution. The practical emphasis is placed upon the task of " saving souls " and the characteristic activity is the revival meeting. Admission to the church is " on profession of faith," and this presupposes the conversion experience. The effort of the evangelist to arouse men out of their " carnal security " and " consciousness of sin " is regarded as the first step in the process of salvation. This consciousness of sin is followed by the " experience of grace." The final result is " sanctification," or the transformation of the personality. Such in brief is the old evangelistic message, which, though differing in details, was held by the overwhelming majority of the Protestant Christians of America thirty years ago.

From the standpoint of our inquiry it is to be noticed that the scheme was designed to produce a certain type of experience and to secure immediacy of vision as contrasted with mere formal membership. It was furthermore a definite attempt to deal with the sick of soul. At its best it sounded forth a commanding summons to get square with that which is supreme in the hierarchy of loyalties and values. To many individuals it brought new life and hope and a character reorganized on a basis looked upon as universal and abiding. It thus set out to trouble the consciences of men, but it also brought them peace and a new plan of life. We may also notice that the great revivals have been marked by the outbreak of pathological phenomena which have given no little concern to men like John Wesley and Jonathan Edwards.[2]

What our patient gets from this group in the way of practical help will depend very largely upon the character and training of the man upon whom he calls. It is a heterogeneous assortment. A large proportion of them have had neither college nor seminary training. Like the groups from which Fox and Bunyan sprang and with which they were identified, this evangelistic group is rooted in the spontaneous religious experience and fervor of the common people. Among these ministers our patient will be likely to receive a sympathetic hearing, and, if his spirit is sincere and if he does not betray the fact that he considers himself the true and only prophet of the Lord, much queerness will be tolerated. In the doctrines in which he is instructed he will find much to encourage and support him, for these doctrines have been worked out through long experience in dealing with persons in distress. He will moreover be received into a group of socially minded people, whose fellowship will be of greatest help to him. In the practice of prayer, as taught by such a group, he will find the most effective possible means of auto-suggestion, precisely because it is not thought of as auto-suggestion but as genuine communion with a personal God. If, then, he is fortunate in the man upon whom he calls, our patient will receive counsel which is based upon common sense, experience and insight into the problems of persons in distress. But this counsel will not be based upon any body of observed or observable facts brought together and systematized by a body of careful workers. Neither will it be based

---

[2] *The Journal of the Reverend John Wesley* (Everyman Edition), I, 169–71, 560–3; II, 478–81, 489; III, 146; IV, 339.

Works of Jonathan Edwards (New York, G. & C. Carvill, 1830), particularly his "Narrative of Surprising Conversions" in Vol. IV and his "Marks of a Work of the Spirit of God" in Vol. III.

upon any careful study of the patient's own problems. Such treatment as he receives will be without any conscious attempt at diagnosis. It is rather in the nature of a universal specific derived from traditional authority. This is applied to all alike and modified only by the insight of the individual worker. If our patient is unfortunate in the man he has chosen, he may find his way into one of those sects in which religion expresses itself in emotional and often pathological forms.

2. *The Ecclesiastical Group.* The distinguishing characteristic of this group is its emphasis upon loyalty to the institution or to the tribal group. It does not attempt to produce an experience or to insist upon immediacy of vision. It has no particular message to the soul that is sick. Its membership is made up for the most part of those who have been born into the fold. New members are added on the basis of instruction and confirmation rather than on that of a conversion experience. The clergy is generally well educated. There is likely to be considerable emphasis upon creed or upon sacrament. It is doubtful whether the peculiar and stubborn Fox would feel at home or find much sympathy among them. It is to be noted however that no other of our Protestant churches has been doing as much in the matter of hospital visitation as the Episcopalians, who belong certainly to this group. The outstanding attempts to deal scientifically with the sick soul have moreover been associated with this church, and I know of no one more likely to be able to speak to George Fox's condition than Dr. Elwood Worcester, so long the rector of Emmanuel Church in Boston and the leader of the Emmanuel Movement.

3. *The Liberal Group.* The liberal group is characterized by its open-minded attitude toward the conclusions of modern science and its emphasis upon the interpretation of the old faith in terms of modern thought. While still a minority, centering chiefly in our cities and educational centers, this group is growing rapidly and would quickly become dominant were it not for the tendency among the liberalized to give up their church altogether. The ministers are generally well educated, coming from our better colleges and theological schools. Among them are great and

devoted men, with wide culture, broad sympathies, prophetic insight, who have a living message to deliver. As a group however they are lacking in assurance. The old message has lost its authority and they are without the aggressive enthusiasm which comes from the conviction that they have the keys to the eternal life. The practical emphasis is being placed more and more upon programs of social service and religious education. They no longer co-operate in the evangelistic meetings so common thirty years ago, and thus far they have nothing to put in place of the evangelistic message. Until recent years even those who were concerned with the psychology of religion were apt to reject with horror the idea that religion had anything to do with the abnormal or the pathological. Of late there is a growing interest in personal counseling, and a number of new undertakings have sprung up in the nature of church clinics, or "life adjustment centers." But most of these church clinics merely provide for the employment of orthodox psychiatrists without much attempt to explore the religious significance of such experiences as those of Fox and without any clear understanding of the distinctive contribution of the religious counselor.

From representatives of this group our patient will be likely to find a sympathetic reception, and he may find some real help, but the liberal doctor of divinity is not likely to know much about the problems of the sick soul. Certainly his academic training has made little attempt to prepare him to deal with this problem. Even in our better theological schools the emphasis is still laid upon the historical, linguistic, philosophical and homiletical disciplines. It is still possible for a student to go through the entire course in almost any theological school and get his degree without ever having made any first-hand study of the human personality either in health or in disease, or of the social forces which affect it. He will not therefore be likely to recognize Fox's genuinely disordered condition. If he does recognize it he will be likely to regard it as a problem for the physicians and not for himself.

THE DOCTORS OF PHILOSOPHY

The beginning of Fox's recovery came, as we have seen, with the " opening " that it was not necessary for a man to be bred at Oxford or Cambridge in order to qualify as a minister of Christ. While the chief significance of this opening lay in the fact that it cleared the way for his future career, it also indicates on his part none too high an opinion of the value of academic training. Probably, therefore, George Fox's present-day counterpart would not make any visits to our American centers of learning. But it so happens that at certain of these institutions there have been men who were interested enough in him and his problem to go back across the centuries in the effort to understand him. It is worth noting that the initial impulse for the study of the psychology of religion came from the secular institutions and the new science had to wait a full decade before it was received into the schools of theology.

One of the first to become interested in the significance of the pathological elements in religious experience was Professor William James. In his *Varieties of Religious Experience,* which appeared in 1902,[3] he ventured into the borderlands of our wilderness of the lost and insisted upon the great promise of that approach. He drew chiefly upon autobiographical sources and considered at length the problem of the " divided self," or the sick soul. As a result of this study, he defended vigorously the view that the psychopathic temperament may be associated with the emotionality which is the *sine qua non* of moral perception. He held that its intensity and love of metaphysics and mysticism may carry the interests far beyond the surface of the sensible world and introduce one to regions of religious truth which remain forever hidden from the robust Philistine type. If there is such a thing as inspiration from a higher realm, it might well be that the psychopathic temperament would furnish the chief condition for the requisite receptivity (p. 25). The religion of healthy-mindedness, he says, is all right as long as it will work, but the evil facts which it refuses

[3] New York, Longmans, Green and Co.

positively to account for are a genuine portion of reality, and they may be the best keys to life's significance and possibly the only openers of our eyes to the deepest levels of truth (p. 163). The greatest religions of the world are thus essentially religions of deliverance (p. 165). In reply to medical materialism, which seeks to explain St. Paul in terms of epilepsy, or George Fox in terms of a disordered colon, he relies upon the pragmatic test. Not in its origin does he seek the validation of any particular belief, but in the way it works on the whole (p. 19). It may be said that in the *Varieties* the two dominating motifs are the interest in the pragmatic theory which James was at that time in process of developing, and the other set of interests which led him to devote a generous portion of his time to psychical research. In any case it is clear that he really grappled with the problem which George Fox represents, and that with keenest insight.

Other early workers in the field of the psychology of religion were interested chiefly in curbing the excesses of the revivalistic mysticism at that time rampant in the larger Protestant groups, and in laying the foundations for a rational religious education.

Professor Edwin D. Starbuck, whose *Psychology of Religion* appeared in 1899, dealt with the problem of the religious conversion experience and its relationship to the problems of education. He used the questionnaire method, drawing largely upon the clerical profession and upon the student class, and thus brought together a considerable mass of material which is of greatest interest to this inquiry. This material, however, is available only in the statistical analysis and the conclusions derived therefrom.

In the cases which he thus studied he found two types of conversion experience. One of these is a spontaneous awakening following upon a sense of incompleteness. This he regards as the blossoming out into new life by the natural processes of growth. The other type is *an eruptive breaking up of evil habits and abnormal tastes by a turning of the life forces along new channels* (p. 158). This latter type he looks upon as *the healing of the breach between the present self and the ideal self which nature brings about not by lessening the conflict but by heightening it*

(p. 157). As conditions preceding such conversion experiences he finds the sense of sin, the sense of estrangement from God, the desire for a better life, depression, anxiety, restlessness, sense of helplessness, et cetera (chap. 5). The experience itself was found to involve spontaneous awakening and illumination, public confession, self-surrender, the sense of forgiveness, of divine aid and of oneness with God and with friends. Following these experiences he found mentioned feelings of joy, of peace, of relief, a new love and desire to help others and a new oneness with God, with nature and with Christ (chap. 10). Starbuck also made a comparative study of a group of cases in which there was no distinct conversion experience and arrived at the conclusion that gradual growth, and that which is accompanied by stress and fluctuation, are but different means of attaining the same end. That end is the emergence from a smaller limited world of existence into a larger world of being and the surrender of the personal will to be guided by the larger forces of which it is a part. The conversion experience, which he finds occurring most commonly about the sixteenth year, is to be looked upon as an adolescent phenomenon. It represents merely a method of growth and of attaining maturity.

Of particular interest from our point of view is a comment which Professor Starbuck quotes from the *Philadelphia Medical Journal*. In a review of a preliminary article the reviewer says: " Dr. Starbuck himself does not apparently realize the full force of his work in the domain of psychiatry. It should never be forgotten that this form of psychalgia, or mental pain (the sense of sin), from whatever cause is the fundamental lesion in perhaps the largest group of cases of mental alienation " (p. 163). The correctness of this observation is shown by the fact that Starbuck's reply is an attempt to draw the line between the normal and the pathological in religious experience. He shows just a trace of resentment against the psychiatrist for claiming everything in sight, instead of recognizing that he had offered a lead worth following up. It does not occur to him that inner conflicts between the ideal and actual selves may have unhappy as well as happy solutions, and that the happy solutions which he is studying might be better understood if they were considered in the light of those unhappy solutions which we term psychoses and psychoneuroses.

Professor George A. Coe, who began about the same time a study of the religious conversion experience, centered his attention upon the factors involved in sudden awakenings and striking transformations of the personality on the part of those who had been taught to expect them as contrasted with those who had likewise been taught to expect them and did not have them. He followed the plan of intensive study of a relatively small group of cases, supplementing the material secured by the use of a lengthy questionnaire with personal interviews and experimentation. In his cases of sudden awakening and transformation he found many manifestations of those subconscious processes which he terms " automatisms," that is, " ideas or thought processes which, after an unrecognized period of incubation, dart suddenly into consciousness and tend to be interpreted as of superpersonal origin." [4] There were striking dreams, hallucinations of sight and hearing, and strange and uncontrollable motor manifestations. Such striking transformations he finds to be closely associated with passive suggestibility. Nearly all of those who had been taught to expect the experience and then had it were easily hypnotized. Those, on the other hand, who had been taught to expect the experience and did not have it were not easily hypnotized. They tended to be negatively suggestible. The conditions favoring these striking manifestations are, therefore, expectation, abundance of feeling, and passive suggestibility with its tendency to hallucinations and other automatisms.[5] He therefore concludes that such transformations are related to the phenomena of hypnosis and trance and are brought about by abstracting the mind from its multiplicity of interests and narrowing attention until self-conscious control lapses and one seems to be absorbed in the infinite (p. 143). He insists that the ultimate test is ever not *how it happens* but *what is attained*. He points out the danger that what is a product of mere suggestion

---

[4] *Psychology of Religion* (Chicago, University of Chicago Press, 1916), p. 103.

[5] *Spiritual Life* (New York, F. H. Revell, 1900), p. 139.

should be mistaken for special evidence of the presence of God or of a renewal of character (p. 144).

Professor Coe is thus led to view with little favor those religious manifestations described by the term " mysticism." By this he means an experience interpreted as possession by or union with God or other supernatural beings. He recognizes that there is a historically and psychologically coherent series of experiences which are so interpreted and to which this term is commonly applied. These extend from spiritism, whether primitive or modern, to what the various religions have called inspirations and to the sense of guidance and of illumination and the sense of the presence of God in our present-day Christian religion at its best. He finds the primitive root of this entire series in automatic experiences interpreted as possession.[6] The method of inducing such experiences is that of narrowing attention and auto-suggestion. He points out in passing that there is a close relationship between mystical experiences and hysteria and delusional insanity (p. 278). The tradition of mystical self-realization he finds to be most attractive to persons who suffer from the sense of " divided self." Strains resulting from recurrent struggles against sinful desires may find relief in mystical practices and the divided self may find unification. The tendency of mysticism is thus on the whole in the direction of serenity, poise and organized will (p. 281). He does not however attribute to it any special value as a method of discovering new truth. It tends rather, in his judgment, to give emotional reinforcement to some existing social standard. While originality does appear in such persons as Gautama Buddha and in the prophets of Israel, the great hold of mysticism upon mankind lies in its practical efficiency in soothing troubled emotions, in steadying the will, and in conserving what has already been approved (p. 282).

We thus see that while Professor Coe has in his study of religious experiences made certain important contributions to our problem, especially from the standpoint of the psychological processes involved, he has made no attempt to explore the realm of the pathological. This he has regarded as something quite outside

---

[6] *Psychology of Religion*, p. 264.

his province and his own interest has shifted more and more toward the field of religious education. If Fox had come to him with a problem presenting so many unquestionably pathological features, he would undoubtedly have sent him elsewhere.

Professor James Bissett Pratt in his stimulating *Religious Consciousness* [7] comes to the defense of mysticism. Without claiming that mysticism is " the heart of all religion," he feels that in our safe and sane and sober fear of emotionalism and sentimentality we seem today tempted to disown the spiritual nature which is part of our human heritage. The glow of feeling, the sense of the infinite, the intuition of a Beyond, the aspiration for a more than earthly life, these are and always must be an important if not an essential part of religion. Even social and college settlements, industrial democracy and international amity are not enough to satisfy the full warm life of the soul. The soul needs a chance for spreading its wings, for looking beyond itself and beyond the immediate environment, and for that quiet inner growth which is best to be found in that group of somewhat indefinite but very real inner experiences — aspiration, insight, contemplation — which may well be called the mystic life (p. 479). But he feels it necessary to draw a sharp distinction between the milder forms of mystical experience and the extreme manifestations. The latter are found among intensely religious persons whose nervous systems are in a state of somewhat unstable equilibrium. Mysticism of this extreme type shows such undeniable pathological features that mysticism, and with it religion, is beginning to get a bad name (p. 339). Between the milder and the extreme forms of mysticism he finds a difference in degree so great as to become a positive difference in kind (p. 366). He does indeed insist upon the pragmatic test, and by that test he sees some value in the extreme forms of mysticism. He does not however, like Professor James, attempt to explore the significance of the pathological.

In his attempt to interpret the case of John Bunyan Professor Pratt furnishes a striking example of what is likely to happen when such an attempt is made without any first-hand acquaintance with

[7] New York, Macmillan Co., 1920.

the experiences of the mentally ill. He assumes that Bunyan's failure to mention specifically any other sins than swearing and Sabbath-breaking is to be taken at face value, and that the unpardonable sin is nothing more than the yielding to the temptation to say certain forbidden words. He attributes the entire trouble to the unnatural theology of the time with its exaggeration of trivial sins and its insistence upon the necessity of the consciousness of sin as a pre-condition of salvation. He holds that in this experience of Bunyan's nothing of any moral value was accomplished. " Bunyan's victory," he says, " if we may call it such, was utterly devoid of moral significance. He himself had in fact nothing to do with it. He was merely the passive battleground between the Esau test and its allies and the Sufficiency verse and its reinforcements. The victory then was not his but merely that of one mental obsession over another and has real interest only as a psychological or even pathological phenomenon. No new insight was gained, no new resolve was made, no change of values was brought about, no new birth effected, no moral selfhood was achieved " (p. 144). The whole drama was one of feeling and all that was accomplished was the substitution of one feeling for another.

From the point of view of our inquiry it is important to notice that Professor Pratt uses the case of John Bunyan, together with that of David Brainerd, to give point to his thesis that the old doctrine which regards the consciousness of sin as a first step in the process of salvation is entirely fallacious. It seems fairly clear that he has hardly the background or point of view that will enable him to speak to Fox's condition or to deal very effectively with those who are out on the battlefront of life.

One of the most important attempts to deal with the pathological elements in religious experience is that of Professor Henri Delacroix of the Sorbonne in Paris. In the *Études d'Histoire et de Psychologie du Mysticisme*[8] he makes a brilliant analytical study of three revealing autobiographies — those of Santa Teresa, the great Spanish mystic of the sixteenth century; of Madame Guyon, French mystic of the seventeenth century; and of Henry

[8] Paris, Felix Alcan, 1908.

Suso, German mystic of the fourteenth century. Professor Delacroix brings out in clear relief the pathological features in these cases, the visions, the auditions, the morbid asceticism, the alternations of exaltation and black despair. He shows however that these individuals were growing in the direction of inner unification and of social outreach and effectiveness, and that the pathological features were meanwhile diminishing. Where in the beginning there were many tendencies and promptings not in harmony with the accepted ideal, tendencies which they rejected and attributed to demonic origin, those tendencies which they accepted and attributed to divine origin grew steadily stronger. The divine possession thus succeeded in triumphing over the demonic. The intermittent sense of the presence of God tended to become constant and contemplation was transformed into action. Delacroix regards the mystical experience as essentially purposive. Its end is the transformation of the personality. The three subjects of his study he regards as persons of the intuitive type who arrive at their solutions automatically by means of crises. In this study we thus find much that throws real light upon Fox's problem.

Another significant contribution to our problem is that of Professor James H. Leuba in his *Psychology of Religious Mysticism,*[9] a book which appeared in 1925 as the culmination of thirty years of painstaking work. This book is based upon the study of the same three mystics used by Delacroix together also with Catherine of Genoa and Margaret Mary Alacoque. Professor Leuba begins with a consideration of the effect of drugs in inducing mystical states and goes on to examine the autosuggestive methods employed by the Hindu yogi. He brings to bear data from the field of psychopathology, chiefly in the form of observations made on the psychoneuroses by Janet and Flournoy. He also takes careful account of the work of other men in his own field.

In the main his conclusions regarding the five great mystics he has chosen for study coincide with those of Delacroix. He finds them to be individuals who, as the result of certain fundamental thwartings in their life situation, have set out to seek the satisfac-

[9] New York, Harcourt, Brace & Co., 1925.

tion of their fundamental desires in the religious rather than in the social world, who have excluded from the idea of the self the tendencies regarded as evil, who have in the resulting conflict between the natural and the spiritual man achieved a certain inner unification and have then turned from their extreme asceticism to a life of active devotion to the welfare of others (p. 188). The mystical states he finds to be important in their development because they were interpreted as indications of the approval of a righteous and loving God. These states thus stimulated those tendencies which are in harmony with the divine will. He agrees with Delacroix that the pathological features in these individuals tended to diminish. They succeeded in overcoming the evil promptings and impulses and, regarding themselves as divine instruments in the establishment of a new social order, their life became one of joyful activity, broken only by transports of surpassing love and peaceful rest. They thus found the satisfaction of their fundamental needs in their relations with God and with the religious community in which they lived. The result was a substantial unification of the personality. Leuba is, however, skeptical as to the real social value of these mystics and of their realization within themselves of the Christian ideal of moral perfection. Neither does he regard them as in any way innovators in the matter of the ideal they came to pursue. This they took from the Christianity of their time, and they are distinguished from others only in the radicalism of the methods by which they sought to pursue it.

Professor Leuba's work is marked by a true scientific detachment and by a masterly grasp of the literature pertaining to his problem. When it comes to the realm of the pathological, he seems to rely only upon the literature. There seems to be little first-hand acquaintance with the mentally ill. He is moreover apparently content to look upon the psychoses, and even some of the psychoneuroses, as organic in origin and he makes no constructive attack upon the problem from the standpoint of psychopathology.

It is to be noted that all of these workers started out about the same time and under the same general impetus and that most of the important work was done fifteen years ago or more. Of recent years very little that is significant from the standpoint of our inquiry has emanated from the student of religion. Books on the psychology of religion have indeed been flooding the market, but most of these are adaptations of Freudian psychology which have involved no original exploration on the part of the writers. In the theological schools the trend has been away from the study of the strict psychology of religion toward philosophy on the one hand, and toward the practical application of such understanding as we have either to religious education or to personal counseling. In the meantime the scientific psychology of the universities has been so intent on conforming to a methodology which it has taken over from the exact sciences that it has lost sight of the great driving forces of human nature. One group of workers thus busies itself with physiological correlations, another with attempts to measure intelligence and character, and another devotes itself to animal psychology. Outside of the work of McDougall, Wells, and a few others, little that bears upon our inquiry has come from the great army of university specialists in psychology.

The Doctors of Medicine

Our study of the experience of George Fox has led us to the conclusion that as a young man he passed through a period of profound disturbance. During this period he withdrew from human society and wandered about by himself in a state of bewilderment and distress, preoccupied with his own ideas and feelings. His ideas moreover were those which we have found to be characteristic of acute upheavals — ideas of death, of world catastrophe, of grandiose self-importance, of mission, of rebirth. His condition was thus clearly pathological. We have seen moreover that ministers of religion are not equipped to deal with psychopathic experiences. Even the specialists in the psychology of religion have regarded such experiences as outside their province. Unquestionably therefore the George Fox of today would be likely to find his way to the medical man. Our next task must be to discover what progress the medical profession has made in the understanding of the religious factors which will enable them to help such a potential man of genius during the crucial period of his development.

1. The General Practitioners. Since George Fox was a country man, born and raised in an English village at some distance from any large center of population, his modern representative will hardly have access to the specialist in mental difficulties but will be referred to some general practitioner. Such a man he will be able to find without great difficulty, notwithstanding the fact that there is today a marked tendency for the doctors to congregate in the cities. The man whom he will thus consult will in all probability be a highly trained man. Certainly the requirements in medical education are becoming more and more rigorous and the group more and more select. The present-day medical course is a full four years of arduous and expensive training, often on top of a full college course, and followed by one and sometimes two years of interneship in a general hospital. The conditions for admission to the medical schools are exacting, most of the better medical schools having from eight to ten times as many applicants as they accept. The course of training in these schools is pretty well standardized. As part of the course there is some work in psychiatry. Although brief, the instruction is in many schools excellent; nevertheless most medical students finish their training very poorly equipped to appreciate the reality of the emotions or the significance of the factors involved in George Fox's religious concern. The chances are moreover that the general practitioner, to whom our patient may go, will have received his training in the days of the old formal, descriptive psychiatry. He will therefore be likely to listen to our patient's story, make certain examinations, find nothing wrong with him physically, and then have him committed to a state hospital where the mentally ill of all except the well-to-do classes are cared for.

2. The Psychiatrists. In the state hospital our patient will find himself in the hands of a group of specialists in nervous and mental diseases. Within this group there is likely to be considerable difference of opinion regarding the nature of his difficulty. Among psychiatrists today there is perhaps as little agreement and almost as much emotion regarding the differences as we find among theologians.

Most of the old-line psychiatrists now doing duty in our American state institutions would probably be content with pinning a label on our patient and fitting him into the institutional machine until such time as he might seem well enough to go home. Their psychiatry is still of the descriptive variety, built upon the foundations laid down by the great German psychiatrist, Emil Kraepelin, fifty years ago. Their assumption is that the type of disturbance represented in George Fox is a sort of disease entity explainable in terms of organic factors as yet undemonstrated. Toward the attempt to explain it in terms of reaction to a life situation, their attitude varies. Some are genuinely interested, some are indifferent and some are impatient.

The attitude of impatience is exemplified in its extreme form in the work of the late Dr. Cotton of the New Jersey State Hospital. He represents a tendency which may be called radical " mechanism " or " organicism." According to Dr. Cotton,[10] " The distinction between the organic and the functional disorders is entirely erroneous and the fallacy of the psychogenetic view can be demonstrated by its entire lack of success in its treatment of the functional cases during the last fifty years. During this time every possible form of psychic treatment has been tried and found useless " (p. 13). He himself during his long experience had felt in common with other workers in this field his own utter helplessness in doing anything for patients who did not recover spontaneously (p. 111). After trying psychoanalysis and other forms of psychotherapy, he discarded them all and placed his reliance upon physical treatment alone. Marked success followed, according to his claim, especially through removal of the sources of " focal infection." He came therefore to the conclusion that we must recognize the physical nature of these disturbances (p. 18). Mental influences such as domestic difficulties, financial reverses and the like are to be regarded merely as factors in pro-

[10] H. A. Cotton, *The Defective Delinquent and the Insane* (Princeton University Press, 1921).

ducing a toxic condition (p. 76). Treatment should consist in removal of the sources of focal infection through surgical means and in hydrotherapy, which he regarded as the best means of eliminating systemic toxaemia (p. 109). Psychotherapy he had no use for. It was evident to him that it was unwise to emphasize the mental symptoms to the patient. Psychoanalysis, he held, would soon be superseded by gastric analysis (p. 185).

Now this view is extreme. Tooth extraction and colon removal in the hands of other physicians have not brought the results claimed for them by Dr. Cotton.[11] Nevertheless the medical graduate, who has seldom been introduced to such disciplines as psychology and sociology, much less theology, and who is thoroughly imbued with the mechanistic point of view, is apt to find such a theory very attractive. The difference between Dr. Cotton and a large number of his colleagues in our state institutions is therefore to be found rather in his emphasis upon focal infection as contrasted with glandular dysfunction or some other quantity X, than it is in the attitude toward the mental factors. Most of our psychiatrists stress the importance of the organic factors. If our patient should fall into the hands of a physician who is radically organicist in his point of view, he would be likely to have his teeth pulled out or part of his colon removed; or he might be kept for long periods in the tubs and packs or treated to doses of sulphur-in-oil. The probability that his problem would be understood and his religious concern dealt with constructively would be remote indeed.

However, our institutions are by no means without those who do take account of the mental factors. The leader of this group in this country has been Dr. Adolf Meyer. Beginning his work in the early 'nineties as a pathologist, and attaining to distinction in this field, he came to the conclusion that the explanation of the "functional" psychoses is not to be found under the microscope or in the test tube but rather in the life situation. His approach he terms the "psychobiological." He thinks of the organism as a

---

[11] Nicholas Kopeloff and George H. Kirby, "Focal Infection and Mental Disease," *American Journal of Psychiatry*, III, 147–9, Oct., 1923.

whole reacting in different ways to the strains and stresses of life. While Dr. Meyer himself has not given much attention to the significance of the religious factors in the disorders of the personality, he has laid greatest stress on the ideas of the patient. He holds that the good psychiatrist should listen with as much respect and interest to the ideas of a deluded patient as he might feel in inquiring into the religious and philosophical views of an oriental. Such ideas have real significance. They spring out of the peculiar needs and conditions of the personal and social situation and it is the task of the psychiatrist to discover the sense in the nonsense.[12] In Dr. Meyer, and in those who share his point of view, our patient might find physicians who would listen intelligently to the ideas revealed through his openings. It is furthermore to be noted that as one of those associated with President Stanley Hall at Clark University at the close of the nineteenth century, Dr. Meyer contributed to the new science of the psychology of religion which at that time was getting its start at Clark and at Harvard.

The recognition of mental factors in the genesis of the disorders of the personality has received greatest support and impetus from the teachings of Dr. Sigmund Freud of Vienna, and in these teachings we find much that bears both directly and indirectly upon Fox's problem. Dr. Freud has sought to explain disorders of the mind in terms of the operation of certain definite mental laws. The key he finds in the dynamic power of the wish and the requirements of the conscious, organized self. In every individual there is a great reservoir of instinctual cravings or wishes, inherited from the biologic past, which frequently conflict with the conscious purposes. Such wishes, commonly sexual in origin and highly charged emotionally, when they are denied natural expression may become split off from the conscious self and form what he calls " complexes." They may then become sources of great distress and manifest themselves in all sorts of psychopathic

---

[12] See monograph on " Paranoic and Paranoid States " in White and Jelliffe, *Modern Treatment of Nervous and Mental Disease* (Philadelphia, Lea and Febiger, 1913), I, 632.

symptoms. The cure is brought about by uncovering the source of the difficulty and enabling the patient to incorporate the disowned or "repressed" tendency into the structure of the self. The truly satisfactory solution is found when the repressed tendency is able to find expression in socially acceptable and constructive fashion.

In any successful treatment there must be a relationship of trust on the part of the patient toward the physician. It is even to be expected that in many cases this trust will go as far as love. If such is the case, it is to be accepted as part of the process of treatment. Without a "transference" no results can be obtained. In such a relationship the physician becomes for the patient a father confessor and to him he must be ready to tell fully and freely even his most intimate thoughts. In this manner the patient is able to re-live his past experiences and to effect a new synthesis. The cure is not completed until the identification with the physician is broken up so that the patient is able to stand on his own feet.

Of particular interest from the standpoint of Fox's problem is Freud's theory of the psychoses as set forth in his analysis of the autobiography of a mentally disturbed individual.[13] This theory seems to shed a flood of light upon the ideas of death and world catastrophe which we have found both in Fox and in the acutely disturbed hospital cases. In perhaps the first formulation of a view which is finding increasingly wide acceptance today, he writes:

The idea of a coming end of the world, which appears in so many of our case histories during the stormy phases, is the projection of the inner catastrophe. The subjective world has gone to pieces. . . .

After the curse with which Faust cuts himself loose from the world, the chorus of spirits sings:

> "Woe! woe!
> With a mighty blow
> Thou hast destroyed
> The beautiful world.

[13] *Psychoanalytische Bemerkungen ueber einen autobiographisch beschriebenen Fall von Paranoia* (Neurosenlehre: Dritte Folge. Leipzig, Franz Deuticke, 1921), p. 259.

In ruin 'tis hurled!
A titan has shattered it.

.   .   .   .

Mightiest
Of all earth's sons
Build it again
More splendid.
In thine own bosom build it anew."

And the paranoid does rebuild it, not indeed more splendid, but at least enough to permit him to live in it. He rebuilds it through the work of his own fantasy. What we take for pathological symptoms, is really the attempt at cure. This succeeds to some extent but never completely. A thoroughgoing inner change has taken place in that world, but he has re-established a relationship with the persons and things of the world.

In the case of dementia praecox no reconstruction takes place. The regression goes not merely to the narcissism which expresses itself in ideas of grandeur. It proceeds to the complete withdrawal of all interest in the outer world and in the return to the infantile.[14]

It seems clear that in Professor Freud our patient would find a physician who was ready to listen and quick to understand. It is furthermore clear that he has furnished an illuminating explanation of what took place in the searching experience through which Fox passed following his visit to the fair. It is equally clear that Freud's theory makes no provision for what happened afterwards. He does not recognize that following the breaking up of the subjective world there may be a reconstruction actually "more splendid" than the one which had existed originally. It is also to be noted that Freud has little sympathy with, or understanding of, religion and religious experience, and that while he might not try to explain Fox's trouble in terms of a disordered colon, he might want to reduce it to terms of thwarted sex cravings. His break with his disciple, Dr. Jung, came very largely because of the latter's insistence that in the unconscious there is

[14] The distinction which Freud is drawing here is that between those end results which we label "paranoic" and those which we term "hebephrenic." The "stormy phase of paranoia" corresponds to what we are calling the "acute upheaval" or "catatonic dementia praecox."

something else besides the pleasure-seeking tendencies — something purposive and forward-looking which expresses itself in religion.

While Freud's attitude toward religion has remained unsympathetic, it is to be noted that he has devoted more and more attention to it. His original theory of the constituent elements of the personality has been modified to make room for something corresponding to religion and to conscience. He calls this the " super-ego." Its recognition has had a profound effect upon psychoanalytic thinking in the last twelve years. The origin of this super-ego he finds in the individual's identification with the father or early guide. His enunciation of this doctrine [15] was followed by an excursus into the field of religion in which he arrives at the conclusion that religion is the universal obsessional neurosis of humanity. It is, indeed, not without value in that it enables the individual to make the renunciations and meet the harsh requirements imposed on him by his culture without undergoing the necessity of developing a personal neurosis. It represents however an adolescent stage of development. It needs to be outgrown and replaced by the scientific attitude.[16]

It will thus be seen that, although in his recognition of the importance of religion and of conscience in the anatomy of the personality Freud has taken an important step toward the understanding of men like Fox, he is hardly likely to see anything purposive or constructive in their religious concern. Religion represents to him the dominance of wishful thinking and unconscious holdovers. These need to be replaced by the control of conscious reason. If therefore he should succeed in winning our patient's confidence he might indeed help him to make an adjustment to contemporary society, but it seems hardly likely that he would give him much assistance in working out a religious message to the men of his time.

[15] *Das Ich und das Es* (Vienna, Internationaler Psychoanalytischer Verlag, 1923), translated into English under the title of *The Ego and the Id* (London, Hogarth Press, 1927).

[16] *The Future of an Illusion* (London, Horace Liveright and the Institute for Psychoanalysis, 1928), pp. 75–7.

A number of Freud's disciples have followed him in devoting attention to the subject of religion. They have however like Freud himself been inclined to look askance at it. Religion for most of them is identified chiefly with the attitude toward the father as representative of authority and with the attempt by means of ceremonial or of self-punishment to strike a balance between the claims of instinct and of conscience.[17] There is no evidence that the orthodox psychoanalysts would be any more likely than their master to recognize the problem-solving character of such experiences as those of Fox, nor the value of Fox's objectives.

Among the unorthodox analysts there are several who might have some real understanding of Fox's experience. Among these one thinks first of Jung.

Dr. Carl Gustaf Jung of Zurich, who was for some time recognized as Freud's most brilliant pupil, developed some views of his own which led finally to a definite break between the two men. Jung was critical of Freud's conception of sex as the basic human drive. He preferred to think of sex as but one aspect of a general drive or psychic energy. This psychic energy, or drive, is for him the key to all understanding of human nature. Life for him is essentially purposive. It has its tomorrows as well as its yesterdays, and the yesterdays are important only in so far as they help to explain or determine the tomorrows. He therefore took exception to Freud's preoccupation with the yesterdays and his failure to take account of the tomorrows.

He also differed with Freud's earlier view of the unconscious. Instead of thinking of it as a great reservoir of unacceptable cravings, he thought of it as including also elements that were constructive and forward-looking. He even held that there were cases in which a neurosis might be the means of producing valuable results. He had thus known men who owed all that made their lives worth while to a neurosis which with its iron talons

---

[17] Cf. Theodor Reik, *Psychoanalytic Studies of Ritual* (New York, Norton & Co., 1934); also Franz Alexander, *The Psychoanalysis of the Total Personality* (Washington, Nervous and Mental Disease Publishing Co., 1930). See our discussion of the latter's concept of the " need for punishment," pp. 202-3.

had put an end to the stupidities which were dominating their lives and had set them down in the place where they belonged.[18]

Of much interest from the standpoint of Fox's problem is Jung's idea of a "collective," or "racial unconscious." In this collective unconscious lie racial memories and racial urges, vague, indeed, and inarticulate, and able to clothe themselves only in symbols drawn from the individual's own experience, but none the less potent. The acute psychosis he would explain as a regression to this collective unconscious (p. 81). Hence the ideas of cosmic identification, or "God-almightiness." Such regressions he regards as attempts at renewal of life or rebirth. Proper treatment does not call for an attempt to cut the patient off from his collective unconscious. It is not for him, as for the orthodox Freudian, something to be destroyed. The task of the analyst is rather to discover what it wants. Correct treatment does not however permit identification with the collective unconscious, but demands a balanced integration of the personal and collective. Fox, according to Jung, would be one who had identified himself with this collective, or "mana," personality and had retained that identification in his sense of prophetic mission. At the same time he succeeded in making an adaptation to the external world which enabled the personal and the collective to find integration (pp. 172 ff.).

Jung expresses frankly his interest in religion. The concept of God is a necessary psychological function of man's irrational nature. The question of God's existence is for him beside the point. Everywhere and in all times man has developed spontaneously religious forms and expressions, and the human psyche from time immemorial has been shot through with religious feelings and ideas. Anyone who does not see this aspect of the human psyche is blind, and whoever chooses to explain it away has no sense of reality. Human beings have always needed demons and have not been able to live without gods (pp. 72 ff.).

Otto Rank is another of those who have sought to go beyond

[18] *Two Essays on Analytical Psychology* (New York, Dodd, Mead & Co., 1928), p. 45.

the problem of preventing neurosis to a consideration of the true objectives of all therapy and of all education. He has thus been led to certain conclusions which tend to bridge the chasm between the psychiatrist and the student of religion and bear to some extent upon the problems of George Fox's present-day representatives.

In his recent book on *Modern Education* [19] he reports observations on a number of children who were brought up under a plan of sexual enlightenment. It was found that in spite of the careful precautions taken to avoid connecting the idea of sexuality with that of sin and guilt, these children were unable to give in to the sex impulse without feeling it to be something forbidden. He concludes that it is not merely the external prohibition which produces the guilt feeling but something inherent in sexuality itself which makes the individual sense it as something dangerous. The child instinctively recognizes that it represents the claims of the species and that it therefore threatens his individual integrity. His questions concerning sex are for this reason essentially philosophical and religious problems. They have to do with the mysterious unknown and with the eternal question of the origin and destiny of man.

The child cannot be satisfied with the mere biological explanation. What he wants is not information about causal relations but emotional consolation and support. This conflict between the claims of the race and the interests of the individual, Rank regards as the fundamental problem of education (pp. 40–50). In all rising civilizations he finds the necessity for an austere and unified ideal formation. This " collective ideology," as he calls it, is personified in the idea of God. Whether thus personified or not, the aim of all education must be to bring the instinctual drives of the individual under the control of the community ideology. In this task the will of the individual must be enlisted. This he looks upon as an active and positive impulse, accepted by the individual, whose task it is to gain control over the whole impulse life. The enlistment of the individual will is brought about

[19] New York, Alfred A. Knopf, 1932.

through the principle of love as represented in the mother and the principle of coercion as represented by the school. Love respects, protects and wants individuality. The state, on the other hand, wants uniformity. In any case, the instinctual life of the individual must be brought under the control of the collective ideal and in this process a certain amount of waste is inevitable. More than that, periods of stress and conflict may be a necessary stage in development. For this reason neuroses, in his judgment, will never be eliminated and the present-day tendency to do away with the community ideology as represented in the idea of God and in religion is creating for modern education some very difficult problems.

While this contribution of Rank's bears upon our general inquiry rather than upon Fox's particular problem, it does reveal an understanding of the nature and function of religion and of the constructive aspects of mental illness which makes it not unlikely that our patient might be received and treated with sympathetic intelligence.

Concerning the ideas of death and world catastrophe which figure so prominently in the experience of Fox and of the acutely disturbed hospital patients, Hoch and MacCurdy [20] have made some significant observations. In the stupors they find an extraordinary paucity and uniformity of ideation. What ideas they do find are those of death and the closely related ideas of rebirth. Stupor, they say, occurs only where death and nullity are accepted. When death means union with God or appears in other religious guise, manic symptoms tend to develop. When death is unwelcome or appears as "being killed," we find anxiety symptoms. A patient can conceive of death in various ways and have various formulations of the death fancy. Only as we take account of such ideas and their relationship to symptoms will the various clinical pictures be anything but a confused and lawless jumble (p. 166). They find in all their cases evidence of mental anguish and they suggest that the abnormal individual may turn to stupor as a means of release, just as a normal individual seeks relief in his

[20] *Benign Stupors* (New York, Macmillan Co., 1921).

bed from physical and mental fatigue (p. 189). The rebirth
fancies, which so frequently occur, represent constructive and
progressive elements. The stupor may thus merely mark the
death phase of a dominant rebirth phantasy (p. 190). Before
an individual can enjoy new life, he must die; and before the
universe can be remolded, it must be destroyed. Hence the idea
of world catastrophe, which occurs so frequently in manic states.[21]
While looking upon the type of stupors which they are describing
as essentially benign, they hold that any thinking which involves
a lapse of contact with the environment is a misfortune. These
stupors being, like functional neuroses generally, flights from
reality to a state of easeful unreality (p. 187) would therefore, in
their judgment, hardly be constructive in purpose. Our patient
would accordingly find in them a certain degree of understanding,
but the true meaning of his experience they would not be likely
to recognize.

The purposive and constructive features of the acute disturbances which bear such a close resemblance to the experience of
George Fox have in this country been recognized very clearly by
Dr. Harry Stack Sullivan in a view which coincides closely with
the findings of this inquiry.[22] Taking account of a series of case
studies extending over seven years, he finds a group of cases,
diagnosed at staff conferences as dementia praecox, that not only
recovered but showed favorable personality changes. Individuals
who before the psychosis had been emotionally unstable, exces-
sively sensitive and extremely self-conscious, emerged from the
psychosis relatively open and frank and with previous defects
either mitigated or overcome.

The rough clinical label of this group would be " catatonic
dementia praecox." They were all individuals who did not have

[21] It is to be noted that Hoch and MacCurdy use the term " manic " to denote
experiences which we have included under the label of " catatonic dementia praecox." A
recent follow-up study of Hoch's cases (cf. H. L. Rachlin in the *American Journal of
Psychiatry* for November, 1935) indicates that the latter classification would be more
in accord with current usage.

[22] " Schizophrenia: Its Conservative and Malignant Features," *American Journal of
Psychiatry*, July, 1924.

recourse to a comprehensive projection of their own problems upon their colleagues, as in the paranoid group; who did not show the multiple form of splitting characteristic of one type of the hebephrenic group; who in sharp contrast with the true hebephrenic did not effect adjustments through the loss of ego-strivings and perverse pleasure-taking. Because his problems are not solved in these socially destructive fashions, the severe conflict remains unabated and schizophrenic dissociation becomes greater in the catatonic than in other types. The regressive tendencies go deeper and it is in this type that we find the clearest demonstration of the " intra-uterine mind." Such states, and early schizophrenia generally, are to be viewed as attempts by regression to genetically older thought processes to reintegrate masses of life experience which had failed of structuralization into a functional unity. They are to be regarded as a series of major mental events, always attended by material changes in the personality, but in themselves implying nothing of deterioration or of dementia. The disorder is one in which the total experience of the individual is reorganized and a great eruption of the primitive thought processes takes place. The presence of bizarre or illogical persecutory delusions may be merely incidental to the psychic reorganization and indicates an unfavorable prognosis only when such beliefs become consistent logically.

In addition to his recognition of the constructive aspects of the acute disturbance, Dr. Sullivan has given much attention to the social factors and the social implications of mental illness. He has not however paid much attention to the religious implications of these experiences and it is doubtful whether he would be likely to help our patient through to the type of solution which Fox actually achieved unaided.

This review of the work of the professional groups with whom the George Foxes of whatever age are likely to have dealings has touched only some of the high spots in their respective accomplishments. It will, however, accomplish its purpose if it brings out the fact that each group has to its credit an important list of achievements and has laid the foundations for a constructive synthesis.

The students of religion are undergoing an important transformation in their point of view and the authority of tradition is yielding rapidly to the empirical approach. The weaknesses which we have noted in our more liberal groups are largely those which are unavoidable in such a stage of transition. Most of these changes have come as a result of the church's own self-criticism. Scholars working chiefly in our theological schools have scrutinized very carefully their sacred books, have arrived at a fairly well-established consensus as to their origin and history, and have sifted out the authentic from the unauthentic. Through the study of other religions they have been released from the old provincialism which regarded its own faith as entitled to a unique and exclusive authority. They have studied thoroughly and fearlessly the religious institutions of past and present and have re-examined the foundations of their faith. Many idols have been shattered and the enduring objectives clarified.

From certain departments of psychology in our secular institutions of learning have come the careful and painstaking studies of those constructive solutions of inner conflicts known as the religious conversion experience which are so important from the standpoint of this inquiry. It has been shown that spontaneous awakenings and the eruptive breaking up of evil habits and turning of the vital forces along new channels may be part of the process of growth, and that nature often seeks to heal the breach between the present self and the ideal self not by lessening the conflict but by heightening it. Studies of autobiographies of certain great mystics in whom pathological manifestations are a marked feature have shown that such manifestations were merely incidental to acute conflict and change, and that the end of mysticism is not feeling states but the transformation of character in the direction of socialization and unification. But it is also clear that no real attack has been made from the standpoint of the student of religion upon the significance of the pathological. It has not been recognized that a consideration of unhappy solutions of inner conflicts might throw light upon constructive solutions and upon the laws of the inner life which are involved. It is moreover to be feared that some of those who have done most in the interpretation of the records of Fox's experience, now that he is dead and labeled, might have had trouble in recognizing and understanding his condition if he had come to them unlabeled in the flesh.

The medical group has also accomplished things of great importance. Dealing with persons in distress, keeping careful records of their observations, and exchanging experience with each other, they are building up a body of knowledge which has led them to recognize the foolishness of treating the individual as an aggregation of separate parts. More and more they are learning to think in terms of the organism as a whole and to recognize the rôle of the emotions and of the social relationships in the causation and cure not merely of disorders of the mind but of those of the body also. Especially have they thrown their searchlights upon the significance of wishes or desires as the driving forces of human nature, and upon the accepted ideals and the unacceptable wishes as the basis of most of those disorders. And some among the psychiatrists and psychoanalysts have been led to interest themselves in the fields of ethics and religion. For the most part, however, those who do concern themselves in these fields are iconoclastic in their attitude and are insufficiently grounded in basic knowledge and understanding. Freud writes of religion under the title of "The Future of an Illusion." Others refer to the "antiquated good-evil antithesis" and talk about divorcing the problems of sex from those of ethics and religion.[23] They propose to eradicate the sense of guilt just as they would the vermiform appendix. There are indeed many who are deeply religious in their personal attitudes, but few of these have made any intellectual interpenetration between the realm of religious experience and that of mental illness with which it is their task to deal. In other words, the area with which the student of religion deals is for the psychiatrist unexplored territory, and for the student of religion the area with which the psychiatrist deals is unexplored

[23] Cf. *Mental Hygiene*, XIX, 145.

territory. The two groups have failed to recognize their common concern with George Fox and his brethren. The two hemispheres of the inner world have thus been to some extent explored but they are still separated by a vast ocean of indifference and ignorance.

A PERSONAL WORD

In this journey through the inner world which we have now completed, it is obvious that we have been following the trail which I myself have traversed. I am assuming that Albert W. and George Fox, as fellow travelers in that little-known country, are competent to report on what we have seen there and that by using them it is possible for me to deal objectively with my own experience and to relate it to a wider range of facts. Certainly Albert W. and I have visited the same infernal regions and have been branded with the same psychiatric label. I am very sure that George Fox also has visited that little-known country, even though the labels were not worn in his time; so also Swedenborg and Jeremiah and Ezekiel and Paul.

That I have succeeded with Fox in climbing to the heights of religious experience at its best, I cannot claim. Neither can I claim to have found among the patients with whom I have worked at the hospital any clear-cut instances of persons who had emerged from a profound upheaval on a higher level than before; it is indeed unfortunate that Albert W., the one case from the research group which seemed most likely to result in a solution on a higher level, should have gone on the rocks. Neither have I myself had a clear record since that first upheaval fifteen years ago. Six years ago I passed through another disturbance, brief but very severe. It is to be noted that this began with the sudden conviction that Albert W. was a special responsibility of mine.

It came to me that this was the case with which I had most in common and one which, if only help had been forthcoming at the right time, should have eventuated in a constructive religious experience, as in some measure my own had done. I have thus little to show as to therapeutic results which have been secured in those with whom I have worked, and my chain of evidence is weak at this point. The theory which I am advancing still rests largely upon the deep personal conviction regarding the value of the two experiences through which I have passed. Even though there has been mental disorder of the most profound and undeniable variety, they have yet been for me problem-solving experiences. They have brought to me the right answers to certain important personal questions. These periods have, moreover, been fertile in all sorts of ideas. They have opened up, as by powerful flashes of insight, new avenues of service and new vistas into the great unknown. Thus at the time of my first disturbance in 1920, before I had thought of the possibility of being sent to a mental hospital, I recall stating that I had come to the conclusion that insanity was the most important problem before us today and that I had decided to explore it. Two or three days later at the Psychopathic Hospital I was seized with the idea that it was my job to break down the walls between religion and medicine. This may seem what the psychiatrists call " Prophetenwahn," but I should be untrue to my trust if I did not bear witness to the fact that the idea which I have since been following out with some measure of success was given to me at that time as by an Intelligence beyond my own. It was an idea of which I never before had dreamed. I believe therefore that this experience of mine, with all its pathological features, was akin to that of the prophets of old. Furthermore, even though the psychologists disagree, I believe that such experiences do serve to reveal new truth.

This experience of mine leads me to look with favor upon Jung's idea of a racial unconscious as the hypothesis best suited to explain the facts not merely in my own experience but in that of the patients with whom I have been working. The experience at the Psychopathic seemed to me that of passing through all the stages of individual development from the single cell onward. At the same time I seemed to be passing through all the stages in the evolution of the race. I was carried back to the period of the deluge, back to the age of marshes and croaking frogs, back to an age of insects and also to an age of birds. I also visited the sun and moon and, like Albert W., I even roamed all around the universe. My conscious self was indeed down in the lower regions at the mercy of all the strange and terrifying phantasms which were to me reality. It was a terrific life and death struggle in which all accepted beliefs and values were overturned, and I did not know that to believe. I was sure of just one thing, that things were not what they seemed, sure also that my loved ones were in danger and that their welfare meant everything to me. Many of the ideas that came to me were shocking, horrifying in the extreme, but even so I can say that there was no giving way to the lower tendencies. If I am today not still behind locked doors, I find in that fact the explanation. Throughout those entire periods it was my best self that was dominant, something strong and deep and tender and intense, which was, I still believe, more than just myself. My great difficulty in the period of "normality" is to remain true to the vision which came to me then. I must recognize that in this present life of active participation in the world of men I am very far from having maintained the mystical identification which I felt so keenly during the disturbance. It is this fact which explains, at least in part, the recurrence of six years ago, an experience whose full meaning is not yet clear.

The interpretation which I am giving is thus by no means free from a definite personal bias. But whatever value it has lies in the fact that it comes from one who has himself shared in the experience of which he reports and whose attempts to understand it have been no mere matter of academic interest but of life and death. It may therefore be in order to include at this point extracts from some letters which show how the experience looked to me at the time I was trying so desperately to find the way out. Among these I look back with particular interest upon the letter to which I have already referred, written during Thanksgiving week in 1920, just three weeks after I waked up out of that first severe disturbance and before I had done any reading in psychiatric literature. In addition to what I have already quoted I may add the following passages:

Now my diagnosis is this: The trouble in my case, as well as in many others, has been due to *a sort of auto-hypnosis.* I remember in one of Professor Coe's seminars we discussed the various means of inducing the trance condition. The principle brought out was that the key to it lay in the fixing of attention upon one thing or one idea. One of the seminar group went home and proceeded to experiment. He fixed his attention upon an electric light bulb. He induced the trance and at the same time he injured his eyes. I take it that when the recent disturbance came on, my attention had been concentrated pretty completely upon a narrow circle of ideas until I had become entirely absorbed in it. Auto-hypnosis is therefore exactly what might be expected. I am quite sure of one thing: there has been nothing wrong with the mental processes or with the reasoning faculty. *Once my premises were granted, the conclusions were all right.* The fundamental fallacy was of course *the belief that an idea carried authority because of the way in which it came.*

I have been much puzzled in trying to explain the origin and character of those ideas which now fill me with so much horror. How is it possible that I could ever fancy myself in such a rôle as I thought myself to be playing in the recent insane period? I see two possible explanations:

1. When you give up everything you have for a certain end and you then feel yourself called upon to give that up, it is equivalent to giving up your life, and your life is for you one with the world and with the universe. What shall it profit a man if he gain the whole world and lose his own life? is a saying which applies. This truth might be expressed mathematically — if my memory does not betray me — by the equation $1/0 = \infty$. It does not matter how small or insignificant the unit may be, if it is divided by zero the quotient is infinity.

2. When you give up, or think you are giving up, all that makes life worth while for you, you don't care much about anything else. Wealth, honor, power have no particular charms. You don't care about them and you know that you don't. Therefore to one's consciousness there is no particular enormity in the ideas of grandeur, much as you may be later horrified by them. I felt that a responsibility was being placed upon me which I did not want and could not stand.

With reference to the particular ideas I shall not attempt any explanation. I take it that in times like this, which are really fertile in suggestions, some suggestions will stand the test of experience and others will not.

I would however insist upon one thing. Most of these ideas were not in line with my previous thinking or experience. In fact they derived their authority in my eyes precisely from the fact that they were so absolutely different from anything I had ever thought of or heard of before and because they came surging into my head with such a rush.

Under the date of September 18, 1921, three months before I left the hospital, I find another attempt at an interpretation of the experience which except for further elaboration has remained essentially unchanged:

I have already outlined my own views in regard to the types of cases which we see here. It may however be worth while to sum this up once more.

I would distinguish in the first place those cases in which the origin is to be found in some physical cause. There is some defect in the blood, a lesion of the brain tissue, a hardening of the arteries, etc. Such are the types of insanity due to old age, syphilitic poisoning, or a blow on the head. With these I am not concerned.

The other type is not due to a physical cause but to a mental one. It is not the body which is out of order but the ideas. The patient's world has been upset. Something has happened which has swept away the foundations upon which his judgments are based. It may be a disappointment which destroys his faith. Or it may be some new fact which compels a readjustment in the philosophy of life. The result is confusion of thought and concentration upon the new idea. This often means sleepless nights and intense absorption and then perhaps a condition of auto-hypnosis in which one loses his way and becomes bewildered. This may be ascribed to a sort of auto-intoxication due to sleeplessness. I am however convinced that it is something more than mere intoxication.

Now I would go a step further and distinguish within this latter type of insanity two classes. Such disturbances are, as I see it, apt to occur in connection with some transition period, when some big life problem is up for solution. In these disturbances we may therefore distinguish between those cases in which the tendency is downward toward disintegration and those in which it is in the direction of the unification of the personality.

In support of this view I would cite Delacroix's main conclusions in his *Études d'Histoire et de Psychologie du Mysticisme*. In this he shows that in each of the three cases studied, Madame Guyon, Santa Teresa and Suso, the origin of their mystical experiences was to be found in an inner conflict and that the general tendency was toward the overcoming of that conflict and toward the unification of the personality. There may have been in each of these cases, as there actually were, elements which the subject recognized as erroneous and unacceptable. There may also have been abnormal and morbid phenomena, voices, visions, automatisms of other sorts, which to the alienist are evidences of insanity, but with the increasing unification of the personality these automatisms disappear; so also does the demonic current.

I would also recall the Freudian theory,[24] which, if I understand it aright, finds the origin of the neurotic conditions in a conflict between certain unconscious forces and seeks the cure in the removal of that conflict.

I hold therefore that all such cases as have their origin in some life problem are properly cases for the consideration of the religious teacher and that the medical man who approaches them with a materialistic philosophy is led to do one of two things, either to give his attention to the suppression of symptoms through force, or else to seek the removal of the conflict through surrender and through the cessation of thought — by the ostrich method, as you term it.

I hold also that there is no line of demarcation between valid religious experiences and the abnormal conditions and phenomena which to the alienist are evidences of insanity. The distinguishing thing, as I see it, is not the presence or absence of the abnormal and the erroneous and the morbid, but the direction or tendency of the change which may be taking place. For the most part those cases with which the alienist has to do are cases of progressive disintegration. The patient is literally in Hell. Valid religious experiences on the other hand are unifying and tend in the upward direction, even though there may be much disturbance and many morbid and erroneous elements. Saul of Tarsus, George Fox, and others I might name are classed as religious geniuses and not as insane men because the experiences through which they passed had a definite unifying function. That after all is the only test.

It is worth noting in this connection that the procedure of the religious teacher has nearly always been just the opposite of that of the psychiatrist. The church has always taught that conviction of sin is the first step on the road to salvation. It seeks in fact to produce such a conviction of sin, to make a man uncomfortable, to make him face the facts in his own life in the light of the teachings of the church and then to square his accounts. The psychiatrist too often says, Stop thinking. Give it all up. And very frequently he takes the position one of the doctors here took in the only interview I have ever been granted since I have been here, that the trouble has been that I am an idealist and that the thing to do is to let

[24] Freud's *Introductory Lectures on Psychoanalysis* had been given me shortly after I wrote the letter of Nov., 1920.

nature have its way. I think it safe to say that the church's method has generally produced satisfactory results in spite of the prevalence of much religious teaching that is unwholesome and wrong.

Under the date of March 14, 1922, less than two months after leaving the hospital, I find the following in a letter to Dr. Worcester:

Your discussion (in *The Living Word*) [25] of the survival of the personality after death brings to my mind an idea which during that disturbed period was very prominent with me. I thought during much of that time that although not separated from the body I was in some new and strange world. And I did not know who I was. I was first one and then another personality, other and bigger than myself. It was a case of the delusions of grandeur so commonly found in mental disorder and the recollection of it is of course most painful. And yet I wonder if there may not be in such ideas an element of truth. May it not be that at death the consciousness, without losing the memories and associations which connect it with this existence and constitute the personality, pass into and merge with some larger personality, the one with which it is most closely akin in purpose and interest? It would be much the same experience as when in some moment of enthusiasm one forgets himself in his devotion to some cause or some institution or in his love for some other person. He thus feels himself no longer just an individual but identifies himself with his country or his college or his church. It would be like the figure of the vine and the branches, in which the branch, supposing it had consciousness, would suddenly get its eyes opened to the fact that it was not just a branch but part of the vine. The center of consciousness would thus be shifted from the part to the whole. If there should be in this anything of truth, then the highest happiness which could come to any man would be to find himself one with the highest personality, which in my thought would be Christ. But some have not made this possible. These may have their part in him through their identification with some lesser personality, some lower center in the organism. In other cases the interests may have been so selfish or so perverse that the consciousness may find itself identified with some hostile personality or it may gravitate toward some lower order. In other words, for all those whose interests had become socialized the group consciousness would supersede the individual consciousness, but the individual memories and associations would remain, and through these there would be contacts with the friends who remain as well as with those who have gone before. Such contacts would explain the providences and

[25] New York, Moffatt, Yard and Co., 1913.

the sense of guidance which all through the centuries have figured so prominently in the lives of religious men. The Divine Spirit would thus be one and yet everywhere at once, taking thought literally even of the hairs of our head or of the sparrow that falls. It would be analogous to the organization of the human body, in which the consciousness is of unity and yet not a cell can be destroyed or a nerve ganglion injured without some awareness of that fact. There is also a further analogy in the fact that the attainment of skill or proficiency lies precisely in the co-ordination of the various members and nerve centers, so that a given idea will call forth the appropriate response without requiring conscious attention. Consciousness appears only when difficulties arise.

I had also the idea that for each individual soul there were two possible ultimate ends. One would be eternal life and the other eternal sleep or death. Pain and suffering would thus be only incidental to the process of growth and achievement. They would cease with the possibility of attaining life and happiness. From this point of view they were to be welcomed and borne bravely.

During all that period the idea of some great Earth Spirit or some Solar Spirit was present. The exact character of this Spirit was not clear but its high destiny lay in Christ, in whom all the finest possibilities centered. But the world rejected him once. It has been continually rejecting him. For me the source of most of my torture was the idea that it was now too late and that some overwhelming catastrophe was imminent. Of course that is past now, and yet I wonder if there may not be in that idea some element of truth. Certainly we are not justified in any great amount of optimism in view of the failure of the Christian nations to do the right thing when the greatest opportunity in all history lay before them. In view of this experience of mine I have sometimes dared to wonder if in the old Hebrew prophets there may not have been some sort of madness in which the consciousness of national danger was the determining factor.

It will be seen that these early attempts at interpreting my experience have remained essentially unchanged. The distinction between the organic and the psychogenic disorders, the recognition of the conflict within the personality as the common basis of the acute psychosis and of the religious conversion experience, the destruction and disorganization of the subjective world, the narrowing of attention and consequent auto-hypnosis, the purposive nature of the psychoses, which I outlined before I had read any books in psychiatry, are still after sixteen years fundamental propositions in my working hypothesis. I have found also much to support these early formulations in the work of other competent students. The chief modification has been the recognition of the contrast between the acute, problem-solving experiences and the malignant drifting and concealment reactions.

All in all as I look back over these early letters I feel much like a schoolboy who after a long effort solves some difficult problem in arithmetic and then turns to the back of the book and finds the answer right. I have no illusion as to any great and wonderful results which are immediately to follow. I am only convinced that in this problem with which I have been so imperatively faced we are dealing with the operation of the most potent forces and the most delicate laws of the spiritual life. I am sure that it offers a challenge to the student of religion and that in the measure that we solve this problem through the co-operative efforts of many men working together painstakingly and accurately and systematically over a long period of time, it may be possible once more to speak with authority regarding the laws of the eternal and abundant life.

On the basis of the generalizations at which we have now arrived we are ready to accept this further challenge. Our next task is therefore to carry forward the results of our findings in their bearing upon the problems of ethics and theology and then in their practical application to the task of bringing in the personal and social life that ought to be.

PART II

THEORETICAL IMPLICATIONS

IV

THE MESSIANIC CONSCIOUSNESS

WHILE ENGAGED in the preparation of our hymnal for use in hospitals I had occasion to submit the manuscript to certain friends. From one of these, an Episcopal clergyman, I received a long distance telephone call. He wanted to know whether I had intentionally left out of the Apostles' Creed the clause, " He descended into hell." It was obvious that to him this was a serious omission. I was able to relieve his mind. I had merely clipped a copy of the Apostles' Creed from the Pilgrim Hymnal without noticing that it differed in any way from the original form. Why this hymnal had left it out I do not know. Perhaps it was in line with the general tendency among liberal Protestants to abolish hell. But in our hospital hymnal that clause has been restored to its place. This has been done not merely because I count it no little gain to be able to assure our patients that Jesus had shared their experiences and thus had a message to meet their own particular needs. I have retained the clause for the further reason that it is my growing conviction that Jesus actually did descend into the same infernal regions which we have been exploring. Only as we recognize that as a fact will we ever, in my judgment, be able either to understand him or to arrive at any true comprehension of those spiritual laws of which he taught as one who had authority.

The attempt to interpret the personality of Jesus of Nazareth is not to be undertaken lightly. His figure is shrouded in mystery. We can be sure of the tremendous impression which he made upon those who knew him and through them upon the course of history. Even today, after nineteen hundred years, millions of thinking people all over the civilized world still see in him the finest potentialities of the human race. But our knowledge of his historical life and teaching is limited to a collection of sayings and narratives, all of which come to us at second hand. These reflect a personality of rare beauty and power, but we have nothing that comes to us direct from Jesus himself. All that we have comes to us through the medium of a tradition of at least thirty years' duration. So difficult and complex is the problem that there are those who consider it insoluble. The growth of the gospel sources is, they say, as the flowing of a stream of tradition, and to proceed upstream, from the latest to the earliest, will bring the investigator to a point where he can go no further. But the tradition itself is a solid historical fact and it is of secondary importance whether Jesus himself actually uttered the sayings attributed to him or whether they were produced by the social forces of the Christian movement and ascribed to Jesus as the head of the cult.[1]

It is therefore clear our knowledge of the life of Jesus is too meager to permit us to use it as a primary source in this inquiry. It may however be worth while to apply to this problem the insights which the inquiry has already given us. It may be that our key will fit. The conclusions at which we have arrived concerning religious genius and inspiration, based as they are upon a wider series of observations, may perhaps enable us to fill the gaps in our fragmentary sources and justify us in taking a less hopeless view regarding the possibility of tracing the Christian tradition to its source in the creative mind of an individual. We shall therefore undertake to consider what light this inquiry can throw upon the possible emergence within a man, whose experience corresponds roughly to the facts which the Gospels give us about Jesus, of a body of teachings so remarkable for their beauty and insight. Can we explain this wholly in terms of the traditions and experiences of a particular race and time, as present-day historians seek to do? Or was there perhaps something new and

[1] Donald W. Riddle, "The Bearing of Recent Gospel Research Upon the Study of the Teaching of Jesus," *Journal of Religion*, April, 1934.

creative, something in the nature of special revelation, as our fathers believed?

In undertaking such a task I am guided by the consideration that the questions at issue in the study of the life of Jesus during the past century have centered in a problem on which this inquiry may be able to shed some new light. I have reference to the problem of the messianic claim. Did he indeed think of himself as the Messiah of the Jews, as the Gospels represent, or was this idea merely attributed to him by his followers? How far did his idea of the Kingdom of God involve that of an impending world catastrophe? And in so far as he did think of it as catastrophic, how far was this conception merely taken over from ideas current in his time? May not both of these ideas be explained by the special interests of the early Christians? Certainly the early Christians looked for the return of their Lord upon the clouds of heaven and they expected a miraculous transformation of the world. Did he himself have such an idea, or did the compilers of the Gospels merely read it back into his teaching?

This problem was brought into very clear relief by Albert Schweitzer, one of the real men of genius of the present day. Schweitzer, writing at the beginning of the twentieth century, after reviewing and analyzing previous attempts to arrive at an understanding of Jesus, sets before us two alternatives which he calls the *literary* and the *eschatological* solutions to the problem of the messianic claim. By the former he means the solution of skepticism which attributes the messianic claim to the compilers of the Gospels and thus strikes it out altogether from the historical life of Jesus. By the latter he means the solution which recognizes in Jesus' messianic mission and in his ideas of the approaching end of the world the one true key which will enable us to understand him. In fact, he says, the entire history of Christianity down to the present time cannot be understood except in the light of the expectation of the second coming of Jesus and the non-fulfillment of that expectation.

The first significant date in this story of non-fulfillment he finds in the incident described in Matthew 10:23, when Jesus sends out the Twelve, telling them in plain words that he does not expect to see them back until the Son of Man shall have come. But the disciples return and the appearance of the Son of Man has not taken place. He then withdraws into the villages of Caesarea Philippi in order to adjust himself to the new situation. There it becomes clear to him that the only way the necessary metamorphosis can take place is through his death. He therefore decides upon the journey to Jerusalem. During this period the secret of the messiahship is revealed in the transfiguration experience to three of his disciples. One of these, Peter, thoughtlessly betrays this secret to the rest of the Twelve. Arriving at Jerusalem, Jesus deliberately stages a symbolic entrance into that city. One of the Twelve then betrays him to the authorities, not by telling where he could be found, but by telling of the messianic claim. He is then tried and convicted on his own bold avowal of the messiahship. After his death he reappears to his disciples in accordance with the expectation created in their minds through his teaching in regard to the resurrection and metamorphosis. In other words Jesus felt himself to be the Son of Man who was to be revealed. He was forced to the conclusion that the necessary metamorphosis could take place only through his death and he gave his life in order that his mission might be fulfilled.[2]

Schweitzer's interpretation has however found no general acceptance. His book has served to focus attention upon the problem, but the tendency today seems to be to take the literary interpretation and to reject Schweitzer's views as altogether extreme. According to Lake and Jackson, Mark is far more a primary authority for the thought of the Apostolic Age than for the life of Jesus. It was written to prove that Jesus was the Messiah. But Jesus himself had made no such claim. The authority which he actually claimed was that of the Spirit of God. Moreover, Jesus did not teach anything about God that was new to Jewish ears. The difference between his teaching and that of his contemporaries concerned three things: resistance to the oppressors of Israel, the fate of the people of the land, and the right observance of the law.

[2] *The Quest of the Historical Jesus* (London, A. & C. Black, 1910), pp. 356–95.

On the first he clashed with the tendencies to rebellion which ultimately crystallized into the patriotic parties of the Jewish War in
A.D. 66; on the second and third he came into conflict with the
scribes. The Kingdom of God about which he preached meant
merely the sovereignty of God regarded as a present reality, or the
age to come in which that sovereignty should be unhampered by
evil. The exhortation to repentance was therefore merely the old
prophetic appeal to turn to the Lord while he might be found.[3]

According to Dean Case the idea of the messiahship had no part
in the personal religion of Jesus. That Jesus believed the day of
Jahveh to be at hand he regards as one of the most certain redis-
coveries of New Testament scholarship. This idea he would have
taken over from his early association with John the Baptist and
from the apocalyptic literature so common in that time. But messianic consciousness had not concerned him. He must indeed
have had an overmastering conviction that his life had been
linked with deity. Some sense of divine commission must have
been necessary to transform an unschooled carpenter into an
ardent prophetic preacher. But to hold that this religious conviction impelled Jesus to apocalyptic self-classification is another
matter. It is unquestionably true that even the earliest strata of
gospel tradition clearly imply such an idea on Jesus' part. But
it is much easier to explain this in terms of the desire of the rever-
ent disciples to exalt their master and make him seem a more
worthy object of devotion. Whence could Jesus himself have derived the notion that he was himself the official apocalyptic messiah
to usher in the Kingdom? What phase of his own experience
could have inspired such an opinion? Surely it would have been
impossible for Jesus to have anticipated in imagination the process
of thought which his disciples accomplished later only in retrospect.[4]

One of the obstacles to any general acceptance of Schweitzer's
interpretation was, of course, the questions which it raised regard-

[3] Kirsopp Lake and J. G. Foakes-Jackson, *Beginnings of Christianity* (New York,
Macmillan Co., 1920), I, 268–89.

[4] "The Alleged Messianic Consciousness of Jesus," *Journal of Biblical Literature,*
Dec., 1926.

ing the mental health of Jesus. His interpretation was at once attacked on that ground by his German colleagues. It would make of Jesus, they said, just a deluded fanatic and psychopath. In answer to them and also to the pathographic studies of the life of Jesus made by certain psychiatrists [5] Schweitzer brought out as his medical thesis a monograph entitled *Die psychiatrische Beurteilung Jesu.*[6] This book appeared in 1913 just before he left to take up his duties on the mission field in Africa. It is written from the standpoint of the older descriptive psychiatry. He proceeds from the assumption that the one possible charge against the mental health of Jesus would be that he was a paranoic and that paranoia is a sort of disease process which originates in a certain way and follows a more or less predestined course. This was not true in the case of Jesus. He was able to win and to retain disciples. He was adaptable and responsive to the social situation and considerate of the feelings of others. He was thus without that mistaken and unreasoning aggressiveness and imperviousness to new ideas which characterize the paranoic. The only reason for questioning the sanity of Jesus is the suspicion raised by his messianic claim. That Jesus did make such a claim seems to him certain. Even after we have made all due allowance for the distortion of his actual utterances by his devoted followers, Schweitzer sees no escape from the conclusion that Jesus did think of himself as the Messiah. But this idea, like that of the Kingdom of God that was to come, did not originate within Jesus himself. It originated rather in a social atmosphere saturated with eschatology. It was thus " dogmatic " in origin. Jesus was one of those who thought in terms of doctrine. He looked forward to a messianic parousia and believed in it so seriously that he sought to translate it into reality, even at the cost of sacrificing his own life. In him we see theological

[5] C. Binet-Sangle, *La Folie de Jesus* (Maloine, Paris, 4 vols., 1908–15).

Hirsch, " Religion and Civilization: The Conclusions of a Psychiatrist," *Truth Seeker,* New York, 1912.

Georg L. de Loosten, *Jesus Christus vom Standpunkt des Psychiaters* (Handelsdruckerei, Bamberg, 1905).

Emil Rassmussen, *Jesus: eine vergleichende, pathologische Studie* (Zeitler, Leipzig, 1905).

For a good review of the foregoing and of the problem generally, see Walter E. Bundy, *The Psychic Health of Jesus* (Macmillan Co., 1922).

[6] Tuebingen, Mohr, 1913.

beliefs breaking in upon the natural course of history and throwing it into confusion by the volcanic force of an incalculable personality.

We thus find among students of the New Testament a fairly general agreement that Jesus did believe that a new age of some sort was about to come. This they agree in attributing to ideas current in his particular time and group. But there is radical disagreement in regard to the messianic claim. Schweitzer holds that Jesus did think of himself as the Messiah of the Jews but he explains this likewise in terms of prevailing group ideas. Other scholars differ. Even though the expectation of a messiah might be prevalent, they recognize that it is a long jump from a general acceptance of such a doctrine to the view that one is oneself the official apocalyptic messiah. Even though such an idea is attributed to him by the earliest sources they feel it necessary to rule it out of Jesus' own self-consciousness. Such an idea, they think, could not possibly have arisen and remained in the mind of any normal man.

It is thus clear that the problem concerning which there has been the greatest controversy in the study of the life of Jesus during the last fifty years is one in which we are very much concerned. Our inquiry has revealed that ideas of world catastrophe and of one's own important rôle therein are distinctive of a certain type of experience. They do not need to be explained in terms of a stream of tradition. They arise spontaneously within individuals who are passing through those searching inner struggles which make either for life or for death, and that regardless of race and regardless of time.

Instead of trying to explain such ideas in terms of a stream of tradition, it might seem rather in order to explain the apocalyptic or adventist stream of tradition in terms of the spontaneous recurrence of such ideas and the missionary zeal of those who pass successfully through experiences of the type that produces them.

More than this, our findings may well make us skeptical concerning the distinction between the sense of divine commission which Professor Case is willing to recognize in Jesus and the messianic consciousness which he would rule out. Such distinctions we have encountered before. It is the old attempt to compartmentalize the inner world. We have found it even in those who approached religion from the standpoint of psychology. It has led them to ignore the significance of the pathological for the understanding of the laws of the spiritual life. The distinction between the sense of divine commission and the messianic consciousness is then similar to that between the " mild mysticism " in which Professor Pratt believes and the " major mysticism " which he regards as practically different in kind. On the basis of our findings we are ready to recognize that a man may make the journey to the depths of the infernal regions and yet emerge victorious. We shall therefore find no difficulty in believing that Jesus did think of himself as the Messiah and that he is yet entitled to the very highest rank among men of religious genius.

In support of the view that Jesus held both the messianic and the eschatological ideas, as Schweitzer thinks he did, we may begin, not with explicit and emphatic statements, any one of which might be attributed to his enthusiastic followers, but with ideas or trends which seem to be embedded in the gospel material as a whole. Such starting points may be found in the following propositions:

1. That the Kingdom of God which constituted the central theme in his teaching was something in the nature of a new world order consequent upon an imminent world catastrophe.

2. That he was sent to proclaim the coming of this Kingdom and had in it a rôle of peculiar authority and power.

3. That he anticipated his own death as a condition of the attainment of his objective in life.

These propositions need not be elaborated. It is sufficient to point out in support of the first proposition that of the fifty-five sayings of Jesus included in the Gospel of Mark, ten sayings with a total of 870 words have the coming new age as their central theme, and in six others that theme is at least inferential. Of the fifty-nine sayings in Harnack's reconstruction of the material common to Matthew and Luke but not to Mark,[7] thirteen with a

7 Adolf Harnack, *The Sayings of Jesus*, translated by J. R. Wilkinson (New York, G. P. Putnam's Sons, 1908).

total of 770 words are likewise concerned primarily with this theme. Many of these are distinctly apocalyptic and catastrophic. It is furthermore to be noted that Luke, instead of exaggerating these sayings, shows a tendency to minimize them.[8]

Evidence for the fact that he did ascribe to himself an important rôle in this coming Kingdom of God is likewise embedded in the materials included in the Gospels. We read that he went around preaching that the Kingdom of God was at hand (Mark 1:14-15). It was moreover a mystery which he could reveal to the disciples but not to others except in parables (Mark 4:11). He had therefore a source of knowledge not open to the mass of mankind, and he is reported as saying to his disciples, " Blessed are the eyes which see what ye see " (Luke 10:24). He claimed the power to forgive sins and this claim excited anger and criticism among certain on-lookers who saw in it an assumption of the prerogatives of God (Mark 2:10). We have also the statements that he had come to seek and to save the lost (Luke 19:11) and that he had not come to call the righteous, but sinners (Mark 2:13-17). These are just a few of the relevant sayings. Any one of them considered alone might be challenged, but together they are sufficient to establish the presumption that Jesus did have an exalted idea of himself and of his mission.

As to the third proposition, that he did anticipate his death as a condition of the fulfillment of his mission, we may notice that his saying regarding the principle of life through death is the best attested of all. Not only is it found in all the sources, but the doctrine which it enunciates tends to make discipleship difficult rather than easy. All the sources, then, represent him as teaching his disciples clearly and explicitly that he was to die, and making their own willingness to die for the sake of the Kingdom a condition of discipleship. More than this, it may be noted that from the earliest times the doctrine of the atonement has been central in the teachings of the Christian religion.

Now ideas of death, of a coming world change, and of one's

[8] Henry J. Cadbury, *The Making of Luke-Acts* (New York, Macmillan Co., 1927), 292 ff.

exalted rôle in connection with it, constitute the precise constellation which this inquiry has revealed as characteristic of the profounder problem-solving experiences. They tend to occur together; where we find one we tend to find the others also. More than that, we may note that the idea of rising again from the dead is equivalent to the rebirth idea which belongs also in this constellation. We have moreover discovered that the acute disturbances and upheavals, in which these ideas commonly occur, arise out of the awareness of danger and represent the arousal of the entire personality down to its bottommost depths and the marshaling of all its forces to meet the crisis situation. Such experiences we have found to be characterized by marked religious concern and by the tendency to make or to break. In not a few cases we have found hospital patients emerging from such disturbances changed for the better. We have also discovered that this same constellation of ideas appears in certain men of outstanding religious genius. Thus George Fox proclaimed " the day of the Lord that was coming upon all flesh " and looked upon himself as the unique spokesman of the Lord to the men of his generation. Swedenborg likewise thought of himself as the man by whose instrumentality the Lord should effect his second coming.[9] Paul's conception of the indwelling Christ (Phil. 1:21) is also suggestive of the messianic consciousness, while the idea of the second coming was always prominent in his teachings. Among the old Hebrew prophets such ideas are characteristic.

That Jesus undoubtedly believed in the imminent coming of the Kingdom of God, that he thought he had an important rôle to play in it, that he looked upon his death as essential to the accomplishment of his mission, that he seems to have expected his death to be followed by a resurrection or rebirth, are facts which assume profound significance in view of our discovery that this precise group of ideas is characteristic of attempts at reorganization of personality both in hospital experiences and in certain men of outstanding religious genius. It establishes a presupposition which

---

[9] Tafel, *Documents Concerning Swedenborg* (London, Swedenborg Society, 1875), vol. 2, part 1, p. 137.

will greatly affect our critical procedure in dealing with the gospel records. Approaching the sources with this presupposition in mind, we must take a very different attitude toward those passages which express the messianic consciousness of Jesus from that which now prevails among New Testament critics. Instead of rejecting them because they seem inconsistent with what a normal man would say, we must recognize that such ideas represent a not un-common pattern among men of religious genius and that they have perhaps a profound significance. We have abundant evi-dence that ideas of world catastrophe do not need to be explained by current popular ideas. And even though such ideas may be current, we may with Dean Case recognize that it is a long jump from the acceptance of such a general view to the notion that one is oneself the individual upon whom the responsibility rests. But if we accept the view that Jesus himself passed through a searching inner experience of the type in which such ideas arise spontane-ously among men of all races and of all ages, then the bits of evi-dence embodied in our fragmentary sources may begin to fall into some sort of order.

If now we approach the Gospels from this standpoint, what do we find?

In the first place we find eleven sayings, eight of them in the Marcan source, two in Harnack's Q source and one in Luke, in which the messianic consciousness is explicitly expressed. These include the Confession of Peter, the Institution of the Lord's Supper, the Trial Acknowledgment, the Discourses concerning the Judgment Day, and the Parable of the Wicked Husbandmen.[10] In addition to these more explicit statements we find some twenty-three other sayings in which the messianic consciousness is at least implied.[11]

Besides these sayings which either express or imply a messianic consciousness, there is the story of the triumphal entry into Jeru-

[10] Other explicit sayings are to be found in Mark 10:38–43; 9:39; 8:38; Matt. 11:27; 25:31–46; Luke 22:29.

[11] Cf. Mark 8:35; 9:37; 8:34; 10:33–4; Luke 14:26; 12:59; 19:44; Matt. 10:28–30; 12:28, 32, 41–2; 11:2–7; 10:37–9; 7:21; 5:27, 33, 43; 15:25. See also sayings re-ferred to on page 133.

salem, of the driving out of the money-changers from the temple, the fact that at the crucifixion the mob is represented as jeering at him because he called himself the Son of God and that Pilate's superscription read, " This is the King of the Jews."

The suspicion that Jesus was not normal, in the usual sense of that term, is further increased by the fact that the Pharisees charged that he was possessed by a devil and that the defense offered in the Gospels is not that he was not possessed but that he was possessed by the Spirit of God (Mark 3:22–30). We read furthermore that his relatives thought he was " beside himself " (Mark 3:21).

In addition we have in three important stories indications of actual crisis experiences involving hallucinatory phenomena. The stories referred to are those of the Baptism and of the Temptation in the Wilderness, coming at the outset of his ministry, and of the Transfiguration, which comes just before the journey to Jerusalem.

Undoubtedly many of these sayings and stories were warped and colored by the views of the early Christians; undoubtedly many of them are individually open to question; undoubtedly Jesus would not have openly proclaimed that he was indeed the Son of Man who was to come. Nevertheless the cumulative effect of this mass of evidence is convincing. It all fits together not only internally but with the larger group of experiences which we have been studying. It is impossible to deny that Jesus did have an exalted idea of himself. It is impossible also to deny that he had other characteristics which are regarded as evidences of abnormality. It must furthermore be recognized that neither Schweitzer's *Psychiatrische Beurteilung Jesu* nor Bundy's *Psychic Health of Jesus* has succeeded in answering the charge of abnormality. That charge can be met only by a true understanding of the nature of acute upheavals like that of Albert W. and their relationship to cataclysmic religious experiences such as we have seen in George Fox. It can be met only as we come to understand the significance of the ideas which characterize those experiences.

According to our findings the significant thing about Fox and Bunyan and Paul and Jesus was not the presence or absence of pathological phenomena; these where they occurred would have been merely incidental to the severe struggle through which they passed. The significant thing is that out of that struggle they emerged triumphant. Their personalities became unified around that which they conceived to be their ultimate purpose in life. There was, particularly in Jesus, poise and serenity and beauty of character. There was a fine adaptation to the world of things as they are. There was the calm and courageous acceptance of a heavy burden of responsibility. There was a mind attuned to that which is timeless. And the explanation is to be found in accordance with that best attested of all his sayings. These men had given up their lives and had found them again, fairer and more filled with power than they had been before, whereas most of our hospital patients would be those who had sought to save their lives and had lost them.

It would however leave a wrong impression if we did not go a step further and suggest a possible distinction between the experience of Jesus and that of his lesser brethren. This distinction is an inference from the results attained in his case back to the nature of the interests involved in the primary conflict. Take for example the case of Paul. If our interpretation has been correct, Paul had been having a severe struggle with those instinctual impulses which conflicted with the rabbinic code under which he had been raised. The solution came suddenly and with overwhelming power in an experience which led to his acceptance of the new teaching which before he had been endeavoring to suppress. The message which he drew from that experience was one of personal redemption. Luther and Bunyan and Swedenborg had also unquestionably a severe struggle with the instinctual drives.

In Jesus, on the other hand, we may see a different set of interests and a primary conflict which links him not so much with Paul or Luther or Bunyan as with the great Hebrew prophets. We may see in him certain striking characteristics which we find also in Amos and Isaiah and Jeremiah. In common with them he seems to be concerned not so much about himself and his own personal problems as he is about his people, particularly the finer spirit of his people as set forth in Isaiah's description of the Suffering Servant of Jehovah. In these prophets we may see men who were good enough and fine enough to identify themselves with their people and go down with them into the valley of the shadow, men in whom was focused the Divine Spirit of the race and through whom that race achieved a self-consciousness which, widely scattered though the Jews have been, has kept them together throughout the centuries. In Jesus the spirit of the Hebrew prophet spoke once again and therein lies the significance of his messianic consciousness. His beloved people were in danger. They were in the hands of the oppressor. He sought a way out and he found that way in the giving up of the hope of earthly dominion for the sake of a spiritual dominion. Face to face with the impending destruction of the national life and of the national hope, the divine spirit of the race which was focused in him gave up its life and became thereby the Divine Spirit of the world.

But now comes the heart of the problem. Jesus, then, thought of himself as the Messiah of the Jews. This idea arose out of an experience common among men of all times and races which is essentially constructive in purpose; and the idea itself is part of a constellation of ideas which is characteristic of such experiences. But what does the idea itself mean? How could he entertain it and yet be worthy of honor as a teacher of religious truth? Does not acceptance of such an interpretation make of him just a deluded fanatic and psychopath, as Schweitzer's critics maintained that it did?

The answer I find in a consideration of the significance of the idea itself. It is, I think, no accident that such an idea characterizes those searching experiences in which the individual finds himself alone in the face of the infinite universe of which he is a part. The questions, Who am I? What is my place in the universe? What am I intended to do or be? are ever central in any man's philosophy of life. Some conception of himself and of his place in the scheme of things he must have if he is to function as a unit in the social organism. In the great crisis experiences of life these questions, as central in the individual's philosophy and theology, become no mere matters of academic theorizing and armchair speculation. The individual here stands face to face with the great realities of death and life, of personal destiny in success and failure, and with the social whole to which he gives allegiance. The experience itself is essentially a withdrawal into the solitude of the inner world for the purpose of getting clear on the central objectives and thus getting a new start in life. And the idea of personal mission and responsibility follows inevitably from the fact that in one's own inner world the individual himself is or should be supreme. He is or should be the captain of his own soul.

But we cannot stop here. It is equally true that the individual is part of a social organism. The personal and social are interdependent. No selfhood is possible apart from social relationships; in each individual, as Professor Mead has insisted, there is present a reflection of the social, and the significance of any particular individual is to be found in the comprehensiveness and value of the social group he reflects and the degree of inner harmony which he succeeds in achieving.

There is therefore in this idea of personal responsibility and mission an important element of truth. Even the hospital patient who thinks of himself as Christ may not be wholly mistaken. The difficulty in most of these cases is not the falsity of the central idea but rather the failure to achieve any degree of harmony and perspective. The significance of Jesus would then lie precisely in the fact that with a true sense of the social responsibility which rested upon him he achieved also the highest degree of harmony, not only inwardly but in his social perspective. This we explain by the view that here was a man who brought to the crisis experience no mere concern about his personal destiny. Like the great Hebrew prophets his concern was for his people and their fate.[12] Moreover, the crisis experience itself was precipitated, if we may believe the gospel account, by the insight of another man. It was John the Baptist who out of his own stormy inner experience arrived

[12] Vladimir G. Simkhovitch, *Toward the Understanding of Jesus* (New York, Macmillan Co., 1921).

at the conclusion that Jesus had been chosen as the Messiah and who laid the responsibility upon his shoulders.[18] Because of the fineness of his own character and the purity of his own motives he was able in the searching experience which followed his acceptance of John's commission to arrive at a true vision of the larger destiny of the human soul and of the spiritual reality of which we are a part. It is, I think, by such a possibility that the faith in Jesus as a religious teacher must stand or fall. Instead therefore of trying to rid the picture of Jesus of all that is unusual and to make him over after the image of the modern normal or average man, we may hold with Schweitzer that the key to any true understanding of him is to be found in the view that he did think of himself as the Messiah. We may then boldly affirm that he was right in his conception of himself. He exemplifies the truth which the acutely disturbed hospital patient is groping after, that man is made in the image of God and can never be satisfied except in identification with that which is best in his social experience. We may affirm furthermore that the heart of his message is ever to be found in his doctrine of the cross. Through him there comes to us the imperious summons to assume the same responsibility which he assumed and to give ourselves completely to the sacrificial task of bringing in the new world that ought to be.

This interpretation of the personality of Jesus is offered only after long deliberation. I am not unmindful of my own biases nor unaware of the common proclivity to read into his idealized figure our own particular experiences and interests. I have however allowed myself to be guided by the consideration that such an experience as that through which I have passed may not only give rise to biases; it may also enable one to become better acquainted with the little-known territory of the inner world, and even those who have not themselves scaled the heights of religious experience at its best may be able to recognize the insignia of those

---

[18] This suggestion I owe to Professor Radcliffe-Brown who points to the fact that this would be by no means an isolated instance in which a savior or leader of some struggling people had been thus appointed and that a responsibility thus imposed is a very different thing from one assumed by the individual himself. Be that as it may, I would hold that Jesus could not have accepted this commission from John with the sincerity and earnestness which he showed, without sharing also in John's experience and standing face to face with the ultimate.

who have. I have therefore ventured to present for what they may be worth the facts which lead me inescapably to the conclusion that Jesus was one of those who have explored the inner world throughout its entire range. With Schweitzer, I am convinced that we will never be able to understand him except as we recognize and accept it as a fact that he did have the set of ideas which we have found to be characteristic of our acutely disturbed patients.

But this inquiry has enabled us to go beyond Schweitzer in the attempt to understand the meaning of such experiences. We have seen that acute disturbances represent a certain type of religious experience. They are problem-solving experiences which are definitely related to those eruptive solutions of inner conflicts which Starbuck has described in his study of the religious conversion experience. They are attempts to face and deal with the abiding issues of life, attempts at reorganization which tend either to make or break. The important question is therefore the result attained. Whether the story of the Temptation in the Wilderness is to be taken as indicative of a period of inner turmoil and mutation sufficiently severe to be classed as a psychosis is of secondary importance even if we were in position to answer it. The significant fact is that from that experience, whatever it may have been, he emerged victorious and that through it he gained those insights which enabled him to speak with authority regarding the end and meaning of life and the laws of spiritual well-being.

While I am thus convinced, on the basis of the facts presented, that the principle of life through death which looms so large in his teaching was for him no polite figure of speech but was drawn from grim experience of his own, it is not to be inferred that this interpretation would require us to see in experiences of the cataclysmic sort something of peculiar value. They are surely to be avoided whenever possible and the task of religious education is always to make possible the steady and unbroken development of the individual. But complete commitment to the supreme loyalty in whatever way it may be attained is, according to this study, an indispensable condition of that abundant life which religion at its best bestows. It is certainly not necessary to prescribe or to limit the ways in which such commitment is to be achieved.

V

THE BATTLEGROUND OF CHARACTER

Two BROTHERS who have been described by Dr. William Healy may serve to carry our inquiry into the field of " normal " relationships as contrasted with the inner world which thus far we have been exploring, and to throw into relief certain considerations which are of great significance in any attempt to obtain a comprehensive view of the territory which we have covered.

One of these brothers had been brought to the juvenile court for serious stealing. His family gave an account of restlessness, of irritability, of inability sometimes to eat, and even of nausea at the meal table and other " neurotic " traits. To the other boy they gave a clean bill of health with regard to both nervous and moral traits. He was the good boy of the household, quiet, merry, helpful, honest.

In response to sympathetic questioning the young malefactor told of an experience a year or two before with a miserable fellow who initiated both him and his brother into vulgarities and into the gentle art of pilfering. How he hated those words! He never said them. The very thought of them made him sick. If they came into his mind thoughts of that boy and of stealing followed. The latter was not so bad. At least it was not disgusting. He tried it from time to time and he " got away with things." He just had to do something when he thought of that fellow and his obscenities. It made him feel cross, impatient, unable to sit still. And at meal times? Well, that was one of the times when his brother said those hated words, under his breath of course, in order to enjoy the discomfiture they produced. He himself never said those words. He wouldn't say such disgusting things. But his brother said them all the time.

The other brother when questioned confirmed the story.

We have in these brothers two common types, types which are encountered in every mental clinic in the country and among those who never come to a mental clinic.[1] They are striking examples of two contrasting ways of meeting those evils which make for inner conflict. We have here two brothers brought up in the same surroundings, differing little either in physique or in intelligence, who are both dealing with a common situation. They have both been initiated by the same boy into vulgarities and obscenities. One of the brothers meets the situation easily. He feels no compunctions. He even laughs and jokes about the new experience. The other brother becomes involved in a desperate conflict. To him the new experience is awful beyond utterance. He cannot bring those fearful words to his lips and he finds relief from the stress of the conflict by giving way to the associated impulse to steal, which to him is the lesser evil of the two.

Now this conflict might have found other means of expression. It was merely accidental that the impulse to steal had become

---

[1] Alexander and Staub in their discussion of the criminal (*The Criminal, the Judge, and the Public*, New York, Macmillan Co., 1931, pp. 54–5) distinguish three types:

(a) The neurotic criminal, whose hostile activity against society is the result of intra-psychic conflict between the social and antisocial components of his personality.

(b) The normal criminal, whose psychic organization is similar to that of the normal individual except that he identifies himself with criminal prototypes.

(c) The criminal whose antisocial behavior is the result of some pathological process of organic nature (e.g., idiots, schizophrenics, epileptics, paretics, etc.).

It is to be noted that the brother who was brought to the clinic for stealing is a fine example of the first type. The other brother, even though he had committed no criminal acts, may be taken as an example of the second type. For the purposes of this inquiry, which is concerned with reaction patterns and motivations and not with legal status, the terms "criminal" and "delinquent" will be used to designate persons of the second type who have become involved in overt antisocial behavior. Those whose antisocial conduct is incidental to an intra-psychic conflict and is unsupported by group attitudes seem better regarded as mentally ill. So also those in whom, as in schizophrenics, the inner conflicts have reached the terminal stages, will not be classed as criminals. We shall therefore regard as criminal and delinquent only those who have identified themselves with an antisocial ideal and whose conduct is supported by an antisocial group.

associated with that which was at the basis of the conflict. The point is that the same experience produced a conflict in the one brother and none in the other. *This difference may be traced precisely to the fact that the one was unable to bring " those awful words " to his lips, while the other did so quite readily. The first brother thus became isolated. Absorbed in horror-stricken fascination for that of which he could not bring himself to speak, he felt besmirched and unfit for the company of those whom he loved and honored.* His very inability to utter these words gave him an exaggerated idea of their significance and increased their fascination for him. He thus felt himself in the grip of ideas and interests which he did not dare to acknowledge to those to whom he looked for approval. Judging himself by what he believed they would think of him if they knew him as he knew himself, he became despicable in his own eyes. The second brother, on the other hand, succeeded in socializing the experience. Giving expression to the awful words, he met with responses which indicated that he was not alone but that others shared with him the same desires and interests. He thus assimilated the new experience and remained frank and undivided within, continuing to be " quiet, merry, helpful, honest."

In the first brother we may recognize the general type with which we have thus far been dealing. The inability to socialize and thus assimilate a new experience, whether that experience pertains to sex or to any other matter vital to the individual's standing in his own eyes, is apparently common to the mentally ill, those at least who are without organic disease. The mentally ill as a group are those who, accepting the inherited loyalties and the associated standards and ideals, feel themselves isolated from those whose love is necessary to them. And the different types of functional mental disorder which we encounter may be explained in terms of the different reaction modes, or combinations of reaction modes, by which such situations may be dealt with. Though this boy was brought to the court for serious stealing he is to be regarded as mentally ill rather than criminal or delinquent, because he is isolated.

In sharp contrast to the first, the second brother may be looked upon as a healthy type. The experience which wrought such havoc in his brother had no apparent effect upon him. Perhaps he had a healthier nature, relatively immune to sex difficulties. He may have been without the " set " or " fixation " due to some early sex experience which, according to Freud, would explain his brother's susceptibility. He did not therefore feel the horror-stricken fascination which his brother felt. Instead of injuring him, it may be held that the experience had the effect of immunizing him and making him less susceptible to such perils later on. However this may be, it is clear that he made use of an effective device which his brother failed to use. To use Freud's phrase, he let the cat out of the bag. He socialized the experience and thus assimilated it.

But before giving him a clean bill of health it may be well to take account of certain other considerations. It is to be noted that he made a practice of teasing his brother. No small part of his brother's difficulties were due to this fact, and no small part of his own self-complacency may have been derived from the sense of superiority which resulted from the discomfiture which he was able to produce in his brother.

Boys of this type, if they develop a fondness for the vulgar and obscene, very commonly adopt a further protective device. They associate themselves with some group of easy standards and they avoid those associations which tend to produce in them a feeling of discomfort. They and their companions then support each other in flippant, cynical, a-social attitudes and provide social validation for interests which their early guides would look upon with strong disapproval. They develop philosophies which rationalize their weaknesses and they rail at that which is beyond their reach. Hence the delinquent or criminal gang, hence also the Greenwich Villages and the Dill Pickle Clubs.

Not even the ordinary social group is free from this tendency. The average or " normal " man preserves his self-respect not merely by finding a task worth while and gaining recognition in contemporary society; he is likely also to have solved the conflicts of his teens by lowering somewhat his conscience threshold. His confidence and self-assurance are apt to be tinged by a trace of flippancy or of cynicism; he is apt to lay great stress upon certain petty virtues or become sectarian or partisan in his loyalties. His business and his pleasures are not infrequently a means of escape from a sense of inner disharmony which leaves him restless and unsatisfied. Hence the intolerance of the crowd. The man in the street is not likely to regard with complacency that which raises misgivings in regard to his protective devices. He may be lost in admiration for the kind of superiority which he sees in Babe Ruth or Jack Dempsey or Colonel Lindbergh. But the kind of superiority which makes him uncomfortable within is not kindly received. The cross and the hemlock have been meted out not so much to those who have threatened our economic interests as to those who threatened the moral self-respect of men. This tendency is to be observed even in the church, the one among all human institutions in which men meet on their highest levels, which stands for that which is enduring and universal in human society. Even here we see the common tendency to degenerate into ecclesiasticism with the emphasis placed upon protective devices, the tithing of mint and anise and cummin, creedal formulas and ritualistic niceties. And nowhere else, unless it be in certain organizations which make a religion of patriotism, do we find more bitterness when the protective devices are challenged. This is true precisely because the church is primarily concerned about the problem of safeguarding the moral self-respect of its members.

It follows therefore that even though by socializing inferiorities serious conflicts may be averted and the personality remain " normal," the resulting solution is not necessarily a happy one. It may merely distribute the strain — or, what is worse, pass it along to someone else. The jokes which bring relief and self-satisfaction to one brother may cause nausea in the other. The unsought confidence may threaten another's moral safeguards. The common weakness and the need of mutual support may result in rationalizing philosophies and attitudes inimical to social progress. And even the group which stands for that which is universal and enduring in human society is itself imperfect, needing constant renewal.

It is therefore to be noted that such renewal comes ever through the prophet, through men of the type of Paul of Tarsus, John Bunyan and George Fox, who have found renewal within through reconciliation with that which represents to them society at its best.

The accompanying chart (p. 148) attempts to show in schematic form the different ways of dealing with such experiences as that which these two brothers encountered, experiences whose significance lies in the fact that they must be dealt with successfully or leave the individual with a sense of failure in his own eyes. This chart is based upon the analysis of the cases already considered together with thirty-six cases of religious experience obtained in a study of the churches and missions in a portion of Roxbury, Massachusetts. This chart has been prepared to read down and also across. Horizontally we have different levels of adjustment. The vertical columns represent the different aspects or determinants of behavior. The first four columns represent the pre-psychotic modes of behavior observed in our hospital cases as well as in multitudes of normal persons. The last three columns represent the types of solution likely to result from the different reaction modes and the means of solution operative therein. The reaction modes of shifting responsibility and of bluffing are thus likely to result in systematized ideas of persecution and of self-importance which serve to maintain the individual's self-respect and may eventually cause him to be labeled as " paranoid." The two central columns represent the types of transition or development by which these end results are commonly reached, the one gradual and the other eruptive. A consideration of the categories included in this chart may serve not merely to clarify the chart but also to summarize our findings thus far.

THE PRIMARY DIFFICULTY

The term " personal failure " is here used in the inclusive sense. It is intended to denote the sense of inner disharmony which extends from the " divine discontent " which is a pre-condition of

PERSONALITY CHANGES AND UPHEAVALS ARISING OUT OF THE SENSE OF PERSONAL FAILURE

Primary Difficulty	Controlling Desires	Degree of Awareness	Reaction Mode	Type of Development — Gradual	Type of Development — Eruptive	Solution — Attitude	Solution — Means	Solution — End Result
Sense of personal failure	Integrative: desire for response and recognition	Clear	Frankness	Normal growth	Awareness of danger or of incompleteness; stirring of profounder levels of mental life with experiences interpreted as manifestations of superpersonal (religious) life; disruption of mental structure and norms of judgment accompanied by a) despair and undervaluation of self (depressions and stupors) or by b) overvaluation of self and unsystematized distortion of belief and conduct (catatonic excitements) — such experiences representing attempts to break up sets and attitudes which tend either to make or to break.	Aspiration / Reverence / Faith	Acceptance of ultimate loyalties and associated standards / Confession and forgiveness / Social support and reinforcement	*Socialization* 1. Progressive unification on a basis conceived as enduring and universal (valid religious types)
						Confidence / Self-reliance	Finding of satisfactory self-expression in social, vocational and sexual life	2. Contemporary and local adjustment (the normal man)
						Flippancy / Carelessness / Gregariousness	Making light of accepted standards / Rejection of primary loyalties and seeking of social validation in anti-social groups	3. Rebellion and development of cancer-like social formations (delinquent and criminal gangster)
						Dependence / Idolatry	Reflected glory through identification with finite leader or love-object	4. Submergence (the partisan, the clinging vine)
		Confused	Concealment 1. Compromise 2. Diversion 3. Bluffing 4. Shifting responsibility a) upon other persons or objects b) upon an organic scapegoat	Arrested: stabilized on unsatisfactory basis		Cynicism / Fault-finding / Punctiliousness / Intolerance / Restlessness / Self-importance	Maintenance of self-respect through depreciation of others / Maintenance of primary loyalties through substitution of minor for major virtues / Escape into self-assertive activity	*Isolation* The misanthrope / The legalist, the pharisee, the prude, the compulsive neurotic / Manic types
						Bitterness / Suspicion / Jealousy	Escape into self-assertive ideation and delusional misinterpretation	Paranoic types
		Oblivion	Withdrawal			Anxiety / Self-pity	Escape from self-blame / Bidding for sympathy and attention	Hypochondriacal types
	Segmental		Surrender	Progressive disintegration		Seclusiveness / Apathy / Silliness / Open eroticism	Loss of hope / Seeking satisfaction in fantasy / Loss of self-respect / Dominance of the unacceptable	*Disintegration* Schizophrenic types a) Simple b) Hebephrenic

effort and of growth to the loss of that which makes life worth living to the individual.

This sense of inner disharmony between what actually is and what ought to be, according to our findings, becomes malignant only in so far as it is attended by the sense of isolation in that it has to do with something that makes one feel oneself despicable in the eyes of those he loves and unfit for their company. In other words, it is the sense of moral failure and guilt which appears as the primary cause of difficulty in those cases which we have considered.

The most potent source of difficulty in our cases has been precisely that which was found in the case of the young thief — an unassimilated experience of high emotional charge. In the great majority of cases that unassimilated experience pertains to the realm of sex. This remains for large numbers of persons something fascinating and terrifying of which they are unable to bring themselves to speak. They never succeed in incorporating it into their philosophy of life because they do not socialize it, they do not assimilate it.[2] It thus becomes what the Freudians call a " complex," that is, a set of cravings or interests which they are unable either to acknowledge or control.

CONTROLLING DESIRES

Three sets of desires are manifest in our cases:

1. Those which find their best expression in the task which gives a man an outlet for his creative impulses and wins for him a recognized place among his fellows. These desires are designated by the term " desire for recognition."

2. Those which find characteristic expression in a man's devotion to his family, which enables him to slave for long hours at monotonous drudgery in order that those whom he loves may live and be happy. These desires have their highest expression in the devotion to that which is conceived of as universal and abiding.

[2] For a consideration of the structuralization of the personality and its relation to socialization see Mead, *Mind, Self, and Society* (Chicago, University of Chicago Press, 1935). See below footnote, p. 151.

Such a devotion enables a man to find life worth living even when all other satisfactions have run dry. These desires are designated by the term " desire for response."

Both the desire for response and the desire for recognition are included under the term " integrative desires " because they contribute to the individual's purpose in life as he conceives that purpose. An equally satisfactory term would be " desire for self-realization." It should be recognized that these desires for response and recognition [3] constitute the social drive, or to use Professor Woodworth's conception, the " social capacity." [4]

3. Those desires consisting chiefly of instinctual cravings or appetites which by their partial and regressive character tend to interfere with the attainment of some new level of development and the accomplishment of a man's purpose in life as he conceives that purpose. To these the name " segmental " desires has been given.[5]

Our cases have shown convincingly the primacy of the social desires. The outstanding evil revealed in all of them has been, according to our findings, the sense of isolation or guilt. To feel oneself cut off from those with whom one seeks identification is death. Man, as Professor Mead insists, is a social being, a part of the social process. It appears to be just as important for an individual to feel himself part of the social organism as for a cell to be a functioning unit in the body to which it belongs. To be cast out is destruction. Later I shall try to show that our ethical standards and values are functions of our social relationships, particularly of those relationships which are to us of paramount value.

The significance of the sex desires, which are a potent factor in so large a proportion of our cases, is to be found according to this interpretation in their social importance. The sex instinct is concerned with the perpetuation and improvement of the race, which is biologically that for which the individual exists. For this reason it is hardly to be wondered at that these powerful instinctual crav-

[3] Cf. Thomas, *The Unadjusted Girl* (Boston, Little, Brown & Co., 1924), chap. 1.

[4] *Dynamic Psychology* (New York, Columbia University Press, 1922).

[5] Kempf, *Psychopathology* (St. Louis, C. V. Mosby and Co., 1921), chap. 14. It is to be noted that the term " segmental " is derived from Kempf's theory of the autonomic functions of the personality and their association with the segments of the spinal cord.

ings which are so difficult to keep from discharging themselves in cheap and unsatisfactory ways are major sources of anxiety and distress. From the standpoint of mental health the all-important question is not satisfaction of the craving but fulfillment of the individual's biological function, considered from the more comprehensive viewpoint. The truth which there is in the concept of sublimation might just as well be stated by saying that a man can dispense with the sex function whenever he is able to feel that he is really counting for something in the ongoing process of race perpetuation and improvement.

Degree of Awareness

According to the view here taken the great mass of mental activity takes place in the region of dim awareness and the task of growth and education is a twofold one: to explore new territory by throwing the searchlights of attention upon what had before been unassimilated and then to assign it to its proper place in the mental structure or organization of experience, where it will either function automatically, i.e., without affect, or else lie dormant until it is called forth by some appropriate stimulus.

Assimilation is to be thought of as both social and personal. We have not assimilated any new experience until we have brought it into harmony with the general social organization and requirements as we conceive of them. To be able to give expression to it in words is part of the process.[6]

[6] A most illuminating consideration of this process is to be found in Mead's *Mind, Self, and Society* (Chicago, University of Chicago Press, 1935). According to Professor Mead, man is essentially a social being and part of a social organism. Human social organization is basically different from that of the highly developed societies of ants or bees. In the latter social organization is based upon a physiological plasticity which makes possible the development of different types of individuals which then perform automatically the various social functions. The process of reproduction is thus carried on for an entire community by a single queen bee or queen ant. In this single individual there is an enormous development of the reproductive organs, while in the other members of the community there is a corresponding degeneration of the reproductive organs. A similar differentiation we find also in the case of the fighters, who are unable even to feed themselves. In man the social organization is based upon an entirely different principle. There is no physiological differentiation except that between the sexes. Instead social organization is based upon intelligent co-operation. This is made possible through the development of language. Unlike dogs in a fight, who respond only each to the

But many individuals never grow up. They do not succeed in assimilating the experiences which are essential to the attainment of new levels of development. This is particularly true of the domain of sex as the individual emerges from youth to manhood. As in the instance of the young thief whose case we have been considering, sex remains at once fascinating and yet terrifying, something of which he cannot bring himself to speak. It thus becomes the " complex " of the Freudians, an unassimilated mass of experience of high emotional potential which gives rise to all sorts of tensions. That such a complex is properly placed in the " unconscious " I am unable to agree. It seems to me to be rather clamoring insistently for attention, giving the unhappy individual no peace until it is taken care of, while he all the time is trying to escape from it by forcing it back into the region of shadow and darkness, or incorporate it into his mental structure by means of some formulation which will enable it to get by in disguise. The root evil is a craving or tendency which the individual is unable either to control or to acknowledge to those whom he loves, and by the same token to himself.

By *clear awareness* we mean the bringing into the open of whatever it is that is causing the inner disharmony. The individual not only recognizes it himself but he is ready also to acknowledge it to those whose love is necessary to him. He is not afraid to tell. By *oblivion* is meant forgetfulness not of the difficulty but of the ideal, a victory of the segmental tendencies. Between these two is the region of obscurity and confusion and befuddlement which characterizes not merely the attempts at concealment and self-deception but also of uncompleted assimilation.

---

other, man is able to respond to symbols which call forth the same response in others as they do in himself. He is able to converse, to speak to others and at the same time to himself. It is possible for him to build up within himself consistent responses to certain common social symbols. In this way the individual takes into himself the organized attitudes of the group. It is also possible for him to influence the group. This organization of social attitudes which the individual takes over is his character. What the individual is, then, depends upon the group which he reflects or represents and the degree of harmony or consistency which he achieves. We thus judge ourselves in the light of the organized attitudes of the group. Self-criticism is essentially social criticism and the sense of guilt is the social condemnation which the individual pronounces upon himself on the basis of what he knows of the attitudes of the community.

REACTION MODES AND THEIR END RESULTS

We are concerned here with the reactions to unassimilated experiences of the type described above. The attempt is here made to bring together the common methods of dealing with them, together with those attitudes and types of personality which are the logical end results.

By *frankness* is meant the honest attempt to face the difficulty and the readiness to acknowledge it both to oneself and to others which is a pre-condition of socialization and assimilation. Such *socialization* and assimilation can take place on different levels.

1. We may have *progressive unification on a basis conceived as universal* with attitudes of aspiration, reverence, and faith. Such an end result involves the sense of fellowship with that which is best in one's social experience and may be attained through confession and forgiveness for one's shortcomings and the reinforcement of the will to do right. The religious man at his best and the socially minded and disciplined man who may not call himself religious but who is none the less consistently loyal to the best he knows are exemplifications. It is the goal of all education to produce men of these types through normal development and without eruptive experiences.

2. Socialization on a basis that is *contemporary and local,* attained through participation in the activities and achievements of one's particular group. The individual thus wins recognition and a sense of social security. This is the adjustment of the average or " normal " man, who does not bother himself about remote problems of world peace or future destiny. Such a man may, like the boy with the clean bill of health whom Dr. Healy describes, succeed in laughing and joking about matters which fill his neurotic brethren with fascinated horror.

3. *Socialization of the antisocial* as in the case of gregarious delinquents and criminals who support each other in pursuits and interests inimical to social welfare. By thus finding social validation within their own little group they may escape any sense of inner discomfort and guilt. In so far as they do not recognize their

membership in the larger group they are not bound by its attitudes. They may of course be active agents of destruction to society at large, constituting a cancer-like social formation.

4. *Submergence,* a type of solution seen in morbidly exaggerated form in certain neurotics who are constantly seeking sympathy and must have someone to lean upon. It is also encountered sometimes in the psychoanalytic situation known as the " transference." It is seen likewise in some individuals who, because of a sense of inward insecurity, identify themselves with other individuals or institutions or causes in the effort to maintain their own self-respect. This tendency is responsible in large part for sectarianism, superpatriotism, et cetera.

5. Under *Concealment* we have a number of common protective devices and means of evasion.

(a) The reaction of *compromise* is especially common among those who would cling to their primary loyalties without paying the price of the complete commitment essential to the attainment of higher levels of development. The frequency of this reaction among religious people is responsible for the charge that religion itself is an " escape from reality." Here would belong the case encountered in my survey work of a minister with an unresolved sex conflict and guilty of marital infidelity, whose sermons were confined to such themes as keeping the Sabbath; and that also of another minister with a similar conflict whose constant concern was correctness of ritual and loyalty to his denomination. These men because of their own inner disharmony were unable to hold before their people the really significant social ideals and symbols without discomfort to themselves. They escaped this discomfort by substituting other symbols. This reaction of compromise through the substitution of minor for major virtues and loyalties is to be found in *ritualism, legalism, pedantry, sectarianism, superpatriotism,* at least when these are characterized by attitudes of intolerance. A man may be punctilious about the tithing of mint and anise and cummin precisely because he is deficient in the weightier matters of the Law. Under this general reaction we may also include the placing of undue emphasis upon merely negative virtues, such as we see in *prudishness* and asceticism. The pathological stealing in the case of Dr. Healy's young thief is also a form of compromise. It seems to be a solution of a severe sex conflict found in the substitution of what in the boy's eyes was a lesser offense.

(b) The reaction pattern of *diversion* is a common and often wholesome way of dealing with a sense of unworthiness. By a resort to activities of various kinds such as work, play, travel, it may be possible to escape a troublesome conscience. This is one of the principles involved in occupational and recreational therapy as practiced in our mental hospitals. To be able to forget aright is one of the secrets of growth and development and work and play may contribute toward this. But it is also true that there may be certain hurdles that have to be taken and that rest and recreation and work may become means of escape. Such is the case with many of our elated manics.

(c) The method of *bluffing* is likewise common not merely among our hospital patients but also among those who pass as normal. There are many who deal with a sense of insecurity by putting on an air of bravado, swaggering, blustering, using big words, and the like. In cases of mental disorder we see this reaction most strikingly exemplified in some elated manics.[7]

(d) The device of *shifting responsibility* or " passing the buck " for one's own failures and shortcomings to other persons or objects is all too common both inside the hospital and out. Its frequency among normal persons can be attested by anyone who has made a low mark on examination or who has failed in some commission and has found himself blaming the instructor or the chief. We may thus find ourselves resorting to the devices of self-assertive ideation and delusional misinterpretation. The end results of this method of dealing with disowned and unassimilated tendencies is to be found in those types which we label *paranoic*. Some paranoic types, as we have already seen (pp. 35 ff.), are characterized by the development of fictitious self-importance. The commonest

---

[7] Not all manics react to a sense of failure. There are those who, possibly insecure, fly off the handle when things go well.

patterns are those representing the externalization of conscience. The sufferer hears accusing voices charging him with unseemly behavior. People are talking about him, laughing at him, trying to read his mind. Scarcely less common are ideas representing transfer of blame upon enemies who seek to hypnotize him, who put bad thoughts into his mind, who play upon him with electrical currents, who try to " frame " him, and the like.

The shifting of responsibility upon an *organic scapegoat* differs from the preceding types in that it locates the difficulty within the individual and involves the bid for sympathy and attention. The famous tennis player, who whenever she lost a match would discover that she had not been well at the time, is an example. This tendency to " pass the buck " to an organic scapegoat is said to account for a large share of the fees which are paid each year to the medical profession. It is seen in its more striking forms in those disorders which we label *psychoneurotic,* particularly in the hysterical and neurasthenic forms. A variant of this attempt to shift responsibility is to be found in the " shell shock " or war-neurosis so common in the recent war. In such cases an individual faced with the painful necessity of going over the top would become blind or deaf or otherwise incapacitated so that it would become physically impossible for him to go. He would thus escape both the necessity of performing the dangerous task and the even greater danger of condemnation as a coward. The beginnings of such reactions are to be found in the child who avoids going to school by developing a headache or escapes an unpleasant situation by fainting.

These concealment devices are of greatest interest from the standpoint of our inquiry because of the light which they throw upon the social nature of man. In the accusing voices and other manifestations of the morbid conscience we have striking confirmation of the view that the sense of guilt is essentially a social judgment which operates within the personality itself. We may be impressed by the marvelous devices and the strange lengths to which men will go to escape the sense of condemnation and by the relationship between mental health and the systematization or structuralization of ideas. The paranoic who succeeds in achieving some sort of systematization in his misinterpretations may be socially isolated but he does manage to keep his head above water.

6. *Withdrawal* is another of the major reaction patterns. This may appear very early. The child who fails in one thing may stop trying and turn to something else. If he keeps on failing he becomes listless and is regarded as lazy. Failure in one line of endeavor may of course lead to redirection of energy into other and more profitable channels, but all too often it results in the reaction of hopelessness. One escapes failure and pain by refusing to hope or to try. Such a reaction is likely to be accompanied by sulking and brooding, and by easy pleasure-taking. The latter is particularly apt to be the case where the primary evil lies in instinctual claims which the patient has neither been able to own or to control. Where this reaction of withdrawal and phantasy-building goes on to the point where the dream-world becomes the real world, we have the type which is generally labeled *simple schizophrenia* (dementia praecox).

Where unacceptable tendencies get the upper hand and the unfortunate loses not only hope but self-respect, we have that progressive disintegration which is generally labeled *hebephrenic schizophrenia*. From the standpoint of this study it is to be noted that such disintegration of personality is characterized by an impairment of the language functions which lends support to Mead's conception of the place of language in the development and organization of personality. Where in the paranoic the speech remains coherent and logical and relevant, it becomes in the hebephrenic disconnected, choppy, incoherent, irrelevant. Schizophrenic thinking is sometimes compared to the thinking of children and of primitive man. For this there may be some justification as regards the types of symbolism which appear. It is however important to recognize that so far as form and sentence structure and social intercourse are concerned the thinking of the hebephrenic merely reflects the fragmentation of personality which has taken place.

Type of Development

1. *Gradual.* In our consideration of typical ways of meeting the sense of inner disharmony it has been assumed that these reaction patterns tend to develop gradually into certain logical end results. We have recognized in the chart three different types of gradual development:

(a) *Normal Growth* — the progressive socialization and unification of the personality on a socially acceptable basis.

(b) *Arrested Development* — stabilization through various concealment devices upon an unsatisfactory basis, frequently that of isolation. In psychotic cases there would be a steady and often imperceptible change in the controlling desires, interests and attitudes until the point is reached where the individual is so queer or so dangerous or in some other way so impossible socially that segregation becomes necessary. In such cases, as we have seen, the prognosis is commonly poor. Such persons seldom go all to pieces. Neither do they often make a satisfactory social adjustment.

(c) *Progressive Disintegration* — increasing listlessness, seclusiveness, and domination of the segmental cravings, with regression to lower and irresponsible levels and with corresponding loss of hope and of self-respect. Such changes are possibly but not demonstrably accompanied by structural changes. They are certainly concerned with emotion and volition and with the organization of the personality.

2. *Eruptive.* The significance of the acute disturbance has already been dealt with. It will be sufficient at this point to suggest that the favorable outcome which we have found in this group of cases may be explained by the fact that the acute disturbance serves to bring the cause of distress from the realm of evasion and concealment out into the realm of clear awareness. Such disturbances often serve as a sort of judgment day, the patient blurting out what before, for the life of him, he would not have dared to say. Just as inflammation in the physical organism is an attempt at repair or elimination, so the emotional disturbance serves to purge out

accumulated poisons and break up malignant concealment devices which have been blocking development.

It may be in order also to recall the fact that according to our findings these acute disturbances begin with the narrowing of attention and then with an experience interpreted as a manifestation of the superpersonal. To the individual concerned the effect is overwhelming. It is a new experience of the sort that cannot at once be assimilated. It compels a reorganization of his entire mental structure and a revaluation of values. Compared however with the sex experiences which are likewise so difficult to assimilate, such experiences may perhaps be likened to an emetic or a purgative. They may be crushing and destructive but they are purifying. Their purpose is to make possible a new start, at least in those cases in which constructive elements are present.

It is important to bear in mind that such acute disturbances are closely related to the religious conversion experience which ever since the time of Paul of Tarsus has figured so prominently in the work of the Christian church. According to Starbuck's findings such conversion experiences are likewise an eruptive breaking up of evil habits and abnormal tastes and the turning of vital forces along new channels. In mental disorder of this type we therefore have a manifestation of the power that makes for health just as truly as we do in the religious conversion experience.

THE FINAL SOLUTION

In the discussion of the various reaction modes the end products were also considered. It is not necessary to go over this ground again. We are concerned here only with those solutions which result from the attempts at reorganization and with certain considerations of general interest.

Following the acute disturbances we may have almost any of the different end results.

First of all, there may be no particular change. The individual may come out of his disturbed condition and become normal again without solving his problem. He may stick his head in the sand and try to forget. He may go back to his former manner of life and to his customary reaction modes. He may continue to compromise or " pull the wool over his eyes " or " pass the buck " or seek escape from responsibility. And the primary evil may still remain. Most of the patients discharged from our mental hospitals are probably of this type, and because their problem is still unsolved, and because the sense of personal failure and isolation is aggravated by the discouragement and humiliation incident to the hospital experience, there is soon a recurrence and perhaps repeated recurrences.

In the second place, the results may be definitely destructive. We have seen that acute upheaval tends either to make or to break. The victory may thus go to the segmental and regressive tendencies. The unhappy individual may pass from the upheaval into a condition of progressive disintegration.

In the third place, he may reconstruct his life on the basis of delusional misinterpretation.

In the fourth place, the problem may be solved and correctly solved. A favorable outcome for an attempt at reorganization seems most likely to occur under the following conditions:

1. When the attempt is made with group influence dominating. Positive suggestions then control and the eccentricities which appear tend to be those of the group. The greatest amount of deviation among the cases of attempted reorganization is found among those whose experience was solitary. Attempts at reorganization are thus most apt to be successful when they take place under the influence of a religious group or of a psychotherapist.

2. When the attempt is made on the individual's own initiative and of his own volition before the unacceptable tendencies get possession and before disaster comes crashing around his head.

3. When the sufferer is able to lay himself bare and seek help from those who are competent to give it.

4. When the life situation admits of satisfactory adjustment. The case is hopeless if the unfortunate hasn't it in him to be something of a success economically or socially or if his instinctual cravings are such that he can neither own them nor control them.

In the case of our young offender a satisfactory solution was reached. Involved in difficulty he found his way to a wise and sympathetic physician. To him he told his story, the cause of the trouble was brought to light, certain adjustments were made, and once more he was at peace with himself and with his fellows. Not infrequently the mere bringing to light of the unassimilated material is sufficient to end the conflict and effect some degree of unification. But in this case the influence of the physician must not be forgotten. It was not the mere bringing of the difficulty out from the realm of concealment into the light of clear consciousness which did the work. There was also the social factor which the psychoanalysts recognize in the doctrine of " transference." According to this doctrine, as it was originally formulated, a certain attachment on the part of the patient toward the physician is to be expected in all cases in which treatment is successful. This attachment must be recognized as part of the process of treatment, it must be utilized, and then in order to complete the cure it must be broken up.[8] This has been explained as due to the fact that the physician becomes for the patient a " father substitute." That is equivalent to saying that in order to help a nervous sufferer, the physician must be for him a representative of authority. In laying

[8] For the early formulation see Freud's *General Introduction to Psychoanalysis* (New York, Boni and Liveright, 1920), pp. 379 ff. During the last sixteen years the ideas regarding the transference situation have undergone considerable development and present-day psychoanalysts would not be satisfied with the original formulation, much less with my oversimplified account of it. They would in particular question the view that an affectionate attachment is essential and that the " negative transference " which Freud recognized is to be explained merely as the reverse side of love. They are also disinclined to speak of " breaking up the transference." According to Sullivan (" The Modified Psychoanalytic Treatment of Schizophrenia," *American Journal of Psychiatry*, Nov., 1931, p. 530) there seems to be nothing other than the purpose of the interpersonal situation which distinguishes the psychoanalytic transference relation from other situations of interpersonal intimacy. It seems to be a special case of interpersonal adaptation, distinguished chiefly by the rôle of subordination to an enlightened physician skilled in penetrating the self-deceptions to which man is uniquely susceptible, with the mutually accepted purpose of securing to the patient an increased skill in living. In such a relationship many phenomena are likely to appear. In particular the patient is apt to invest the physician with the attributes of those he has known in the past who have been for him representatives of authority. Hence the attitudes of affection. Hence also those of hostility. The one attitude is quite as favorable to successful treatment as the other, provided only the patient is willing to discuss them with the physician. In fact some excellent psychoanalysts center the entire treatment around a frank consideration of the origin and meaning of the patient's attitudes toward them. It is to be noted however that the changing conceptions of the transference relationship tend rather to enhance its social significance and that release from the sense of isolation (estrangement) and the attainment of autonomy (maturity) remain still the goals of psychoanalytic procedure.

bare to the physician his inner difficulties, the patient places himself at the bar of judgment and gives to the physician power to bind or loose. If the physician, after hearing the story and knowing the worst, does not condemn, he may feel himself restored to right relationship with those whose love is necessary to him. He may feel himself forgiven and able to meet his fellows with his head up and hope in his heart. And in saying that before the process of cure is complete the transference relationship must be broken up, Freud has recognized that no solution involving an attitude of submergence can be a satisfactory one. No man can be dependent upon another human being, whether physician or mother or wife, and yet be free and well. The structure of the personality must be built upon the enduring foundation represented by true religion. The individual, as Professor Mead points out, must learn to respond to that to which others also respond (see footnote, p. 151). Such a common object of response is best found in the supreme loyalty which in most men and in most societies is represented in their idea of God. Of this I shall speak in the next chapter.

According to this view no solution which does not involve progressive socialization and unification on a basis conceived as universal and abiding can ever be permanently satisfactory. It is not sufficient to be free from inner conflict. Judged by the standards of the good which is ever in the process of becoming, which is not yet but ought to be, the one brother may have been in no happier state than the other. The very complacency which gave him a clean bill of health in the eyes of his family may be as the carefree unconcern of the animal. It may be even an obstacle in the path of progress. Only time will tell and the understanding which is based upon all the facts after the adventure of life is completed. The ultimate test is the biological test, the test of survival — stated, however, not in terms of the individual but of society as a whole and the more abundant life which ought to be achieved. Therefore I say that the only truly satisfactory solution is one which results in progressive unification with the fellowship which has the capacity for universality. But this proposition will require another chapter.

VI

THE PROBLEM OF RIGHT AND WRONG

IN AN ILLUMINATING discussion of the psychiatric aspect of delinquency [1] Dr. Abraham Myerson, after describing the unorganized character of the industrial, social, sexual and emotional life of delinquents, interjects the following remark:

> In using the terms "organized" and "unorganized," especially in relation to sex, there is no moral connotation. There is no pretence to praise or blame, nor any effort to set up good or bad ethical standards, to say that one kind of conduct is higher or lower than another. The degree of social evolution in the organization is alone taken into account.

He goes on to say that delinquents are unorganized in their sexual life as well as in their industrial career. Even when married, there is no sense of sentiment or of responsibility. They are never heroes of tense love dreams, of sacrifice for a woman's love. With them love is merely an appetite to be satisfied; when it is satisfied, the object by which it is satisfied is forgotten. Woman as an occasional playmate appeals to them. Woman as someone to work for, to make sacrifices for, to live with in anything like companionship has no meaning for them. Their sexual activity never becomes merged with the mores and thus socialized. Their sexuality does not evolve into responsibility and sentiment. It thus remains unorganized and they themselves are unevolved individuals. In their social life he finds them gregarious without any communal feeling. They must be with others and are uneasy when alone, but there is no deep concern for those whom they meet, no loyalty to

[1] *American Journal of Psychiatry,* Nov., 1933.

men or cause. Emotionally there is no brooding over the past, no fervent building for the future. Their emotional life is shallow, though often violent enough for a short period of time. Their mood is that which suits the moment. They have never built up in their lives substantial purposes which will weather the vagrant urges of the present moment. They are thus in their emotional life unorganized. They have never attained to adult development.

This interjected remark of Dr. Myerson's is representative of a widespread attitude among psychiatrists and others of the humanistic scientists. They profess unconcern over the problem of right and wrong. Among them a prevalent point of view identifies the *normal* with the *average* and some even talk with condescending superiority about "the antiquated good-evil antithesis." Such scientists take the position that their task is merely to observe with cold detachment and to record the results of their observations according to the norms of greatest frequency. Intelligence, whatever it may be, is thus measured in terms of averages, and among medical men the term "pathological" is defined as any deviation from the average. Even though that deviation may be useful, some would say it is still pathological,[2] for the value judgment is not within the province of the biologist. It is therefore not to be wondered at that when medical men turn their attention to the field of human character, as in psychiatry they do, they make use of the same yardstick. The normal is what most people do, and any deviation from the normal they look upon with suspicion and disfavor. Most people have their share of human frailty. A measure of human frailty is therefore normal and to say that a person is very conscientious is not praise. To be good is unusual and therefore abnormal. A prominent lecturer on mental health thus talks about eradicating the sense of guilt just as he would a vermiform appendix. By this he apparently means not that what we call sin is an anachronism, a mode of behavior which once was useful but now is so no longer, but rather, if I understand him

---

[2] See article on "Pathology" in the *Encyclopedia Britannica,* 11th edition, for an emphatic statement of this position.

aright, that conscience itself is as an outgrown appendix and ought to be subjected to the psychoanalytic scalpel.

But the medical man does not hold consistently to such a view of what is normative. I was interested to observe that a certain hospital superintendent, who inclines to the usual medical attitude, took a very different position with reference to the standards of mental hospitals when he was made chairman of the committee concerned therewith. He was interested in grading up and raising the existing standards. In pursuance of his task he took as his norm the best he could find and introduced a value judgment which he applied quite rigorously.

The same observation I made years ago during the time when my lot was cast among professional foresters. There also we used the term "normal" in two different senses. When we were merely observing, the average was our norm. We thus determined the volume and shape of the white pine by measuring up several thousand trees and taking the average. Not so when we were proposing to raise crops of timber. The normal forest was the type of forest we sought to produce, the forest with fully stocked stands and proper distribution of age classes, such as would produce the maximum sustained yield. When I was sent out to construct a yield table for white pine, my instructions were to select the very best stands I could find and to make allowance for "fail places." Any particular woodlot we proposed to grade in terms of this ideal stand.

These two observations point to a very definite conclusion. What for us is normative, or "normal," is determined by our point of view. *If we are merely detached observers or are content to take things as they are, we use the term normal in the sense of average.* But just as soon as we become interested in accomplishing something, *as soon as we cease to be mere observers and become participants in some enterprise, then our objective becomes for us the normative* and we introduce the value-judgment. In some form or other we use the "good-bad antithesis."

Now Dr. Myerson is by no means a mere detached observer. He is a psychiatrist and not a bad one at that. He is thus concerned in helping the unadjusted to make more satisfactory adjustments. We need not be surprised therefore to observe that in spite of his disclaimer, he does introduce the value-judgment. Like the biologist who denies all concern with value-judgments and yet talks about " higher " and " lower " animals, like the social worker who scorns the idea of " sin " and yet refers to " maladjustments," he talks about the " organized " and the " unorganized," about " maturity " and " immaturity." He merely replaces the familiar words " good " and " bad " by new terms.

We are therefore hardly ready to take at face value Dr. Myerson's disclaimer of any concern with ethical standards. We may on the contrary recognize that he makes a very real contribution to that problem in his distinction between the organized and the unorganized. By means of his observations of certain types of persons he provides a basis for a more intelligent understanding of what constitutes good and bad. That, I take it, is one of our great needs today, to provide through empirical observation and tested experience a basis for our generalizations regarding those types of conduct which make for the richer and more abundant personal and social life.

Nowhere better than in a mental hospital do we have such an opportunity. In the majority of the cases which come to us each year the causative factors are not to be found in demonstrable organic disease. The difficulty is rather in the realm of emotion and volition, of belief and attitude. We are dealing with individuals whose behavior is guided and controlled by certain desires and value-judgments. We see these individuals breaking or broken under the stresses and strains of love and hate and fear and anger. We see them grappling with the issues of spiritual life and death, of survival and destruction; and we are able to observe the end results of the diverse ways in which individuals deal with failure to measure up to the moral standards which they have accepted as their own. In these end results we see in exaggerated form processes which are present in health together with their logical outcome. If, therefore, we have eyes to see and wisdom to interpret, we may be able to discover the laws which

have to do with the attainment of the moral objectives of particular individuals. We may be able to throw some light upon the factors which enter into the determination of these objectives and of
their associated hierarchy of values. And we may be able to draw
some conclusions in regard to the social implications and consequences of different types of moral objectives and ethical systems.

A particular case may serve as an illustration and point of de-
parture for some generalizations concerning the problem of good
and evil which have been arrived at through this inquiry.

James G., a grocery clerk of twenty-nine years, with ninth grade
education, fair intelligence, good physique and without organic
disease, was brought to the hospital in an acutely disturbed condition. From the patient himself, and from his relatives, the following facts were learned regarding his life: He was born in the
home of a southern clergyman, who died when he was twelve
years old. As a boy he had certain difficulties in learning to manage
his sex drive. At the age of sixteen he left home without having
reached any solution of this problem and fared forth into the
great world, finally landing in the army. Here he stayed nine
years, making a fairly good adjustment and serving most of his
time as a noncommissioned officer. In the army, along with the
majority of his mates, he found an outlet for the troublesome sex
drive by going to houses of prostitution. Inasmuch as such conduct was sanctioned by the group opinion, he was quite comfortable about his manner of life, especially in view of the fact that he
was always careful to report after each indulgence and get his
prophylactic treatment and the protection against disease which
this insured. At the end of the nine years he married and in due
course of time a child arrived. With the birth of the child came a
mental disturbance, something which happens sometimes to
fathers as well as to mothers. To use his own words, there was
something funny about the way his child was born. When the
news came, his mind began running and jumping. A million
things were passing through his head. He was under a spell of
fear. He felt that he had a lot of responsibility, but he wasn't thinking so much about the baby. He was thinking about human na-

ture and its mechanisms.   He was trying to understand what was the cause of all emotion and he wrote an article expounding his theory of the human emotions.   This he sent to a local newspaper and he took great satisfaction in the fact that it was published.

This disturbance gradually subsided and he remained well until things began to go wrong with him economically.   He set up in business for himself and was burned out.   He obtained and lost several jobs.   He became involved in debt.   Then he broke mentally once more; as at the time of the birth of his child, he became concerned about cosmic affairs.   When he came to the hospital he told the following story:

How did it start?   I hardly know.   I think it was the smell of the fish. I had dreams of crawling along the bottom of the sea among the fish and the oysters and everything.   I had to give up work and sit around and brood.   Then ideas came to me.   I didn't have to search for words.   It was just as if I had been commanded to say certain words I had never heard of before.   I had a vision and it seemed as if I could see way back to the beginning of all creation.   I could see the evolution of man up to his present being.   And then it came to me that from the beginning of the world there have been two rulers over the people of the world, God and Satan.   One was just as powerful as the other.   It seemed to me that a greater effort should be made so that both should become one.   God should be brought forth to meet Satan and then Satan could go and teach the people the right.   Of course this would take years and years.   It was to be my job to start it and to get the spirit working.   It was my vision that in time all humanity would love absolutely and perfectly and without any nourishment and that God intended all people to be just one living piece of humanity.   The church would continue but it would have to draw under one heading, that is, under the teachings.   Yes, of course, that will be what I call the millennium, that is, all humanity striving to reach for one goal and for the kingdom of heaven.

You see, it has always been my nature to do right.   There has been a lot of talk about this thing and that thing, about the farm problem and so on.   It was my idea that I could see no earthly reason for some of these animals that were roaming around in the forests, preying upon the domesticated animals.   I thought it would be just the thing to go back to the jungles and clean up the snakes and the alligators and the reptiles.

Yes, I have always been a thinker.   I have read about some of our famous characters.   I have also read fiction and vice and have indulged in all the little things of life. I have always been a double personality. I have had two consciences.

You see, I interpret it that there has always been a battle between the two for supremacy. I could see no earthly reason why such a conflict should be kept up. I didn't see why the Lord intended that people should be always and forever fighting each other. Thinking it was the true light of God, it seemed to me that in some way I might bring this to Satan's attention, so that he could bring all his following into the light. It is my belief that people of the Protestant faith — well, I must bring it back to myself. I am the true spirit of God and the product of the earliest stages of man after it was evolved from the seas. When I was in the rage there was something telling me that I was the true spirit of Christ.

Rather a grotesque set of ideas! And yet, as we have already seen, they are thoroughly typical of acute disturbances. They also have a meaning and the task of the psychiatrist, in the words of Dr. Adolf Meyer, is to discover the sense in the nonsense.

For the purpose of this study the first thing to notice is the marked religious concern which the patient showed. Each of the two disturbances began with the sense of mystery. It was the idea that there was something strange about the way his baby was born which set his mind running and jumping. And in the second disturbance ideas came to him which he had never before heard and with which he himself seemed to have nothing to do. We notice that he goes on to concern himself with cosmic affairs and that he personalizes the forces which he conceives to be in control. We have encountered this in other cases of acute disturbance and upheaval. Such cases begin almost invariably with an eruption of the lower strata of consciousness which is interpreted as a manifestation of the superpersonal. To the individual concerned the effect is overwhelming. It shatters the foundations of his mental structure. It sweeps him away from his moorings out into the uncharted seas of the inner world. He is no longer concerned about the merely individual, but about the cosmic and the universal. Very commonly he thinks of himself as in the central rôle in the cosmic drama. Such experiences are as old as the human race. Their destructive effects led to the ancient question, " Can a man see God and live? " We have found however that their effects are by no means always destructive, and we have come to the conclusion that they are essentially attempts at reorganization in which the entire personality is aroused and its forces marshaled to meet some serious obstacle to growth. Our figures show that these emotional upheavals make for change either for the better or for the worse. In contrast to cases characterized by a gradual onset and by a lesser degree of disturbance, acute disturbances show a large proportion of cases in which the patients go out of the hospital completely recovered or else find their way to the back wards as hopeless wrecks. Such experiences are, as we have seen, closely related to those of such outstanding religious geniuses as John Bunyan, George Fox, Emanuel Swedenborg and Saul of Tarsus, who through just such ordeals found the end and meaning of their lives. Even though the outcome be disastrous, experiences of this type are religious experiences in that the individuals who pass through them agree in feeling themselves in touch with some mighty personal force to which generally they give the name of God. From the standpoint of our inquiry the important point is the terrific impact of the idea with which the disturbance begins and the tendency to think of the ultimate realities of life in personal terms. When we see the results of such experiences in lives destroyed or in lives made over and sent forth sometimes into new and creative work, the suggestion comes that of all human needs the deepest and most fundamental is that for response and approval by that social something which is symbolized by the term God, and that this fact has important implications for the social sciences as well as for psychiatry and psychology. These implications may become more apparent if we consider the significance of our patient's interesting proposal to bring about an understanding between God and Satan.

In reviewing our patient's history we may notice first of all that he was born and reared in a religious home. His father was a clergyman of the ultraconservative type and his mother a devoted church worker. From childhood on, he tells us, it had always been his nature to do right. That is, he accepted without question the teachings of his parents and of the church to which they belonged. But he had also been " a double personality." This means that, while wanting to conform to the parental teachings, he found within himself certain difficulties which he was unable to resolve in accordance with their standards. There were certain instinctual outcroppings which he was unable either to own or to control and which therefore remained unassimilated. At the age of sixteen he left home and after a short period of wanderings he enlisted in the army. He not only put on the uniform, but with it he accepted also its easier standards of sex morality. Supported now by the group and its attitudes he was able to give expression to the troublesome sex drive and to be quite frank and comfortable about it. He seemed thus to have made a real adjustment. But with his marriage and then with the birth of his child, the situation changed. It was no longer sufficient for him to feel himself a member of the army group. The responsibilities of parenthood identified him once more with his own father and with his other early guides and their teachings. He began now to think of his father's God, the symbol of his primary group and of his primary loyalty, whose authority he had never questioned but from whom he had run away. It is quite clear that measured by the organized attitudes of his primary group [3] he would be found wanting.[4] But

[3] Cf. C. H. Cooley, "Human nature is not something existing separately in the individual, but a *group-nature or primary phase of society*. . . . It is the nature which is developed and expressed in those simple, face to face groups that are somewhat alike in all societies, groups of the family, the playground, the neighborhood. In the essential similarity of these is to be found the basis, in experience, for similar ideas and sentiments in the human mind. In these, everywhere, human nature comes into existence." *Social Organization* (New York, Charles Scribner's Sons, 1909), p. 30.

[4] Cf. John Dewey: " When a child acts, those about him react. They shower encouragement upon him, visit him with approval, or they bestow frowns and rebukes. What others do to us when we act is as natural a consequence of our action as what the fire does to us when we plunge our hands in it. . . . In language and imagination we rehearse the responses of others just as we dramatically enact other consequences. We foreknow how others will act, and the foreknowledge is the beginning of judgment passed on the action. We know *with* them; there is conscience. An assembly is formed within our breast which discusses and appraises proposed and performed acts. The community without becomes a forum and tribunal within, a judgment seat of charges, assessments and exculpations. Our thoughts of our own actions are saturated with the ideas that others entertain about them, ideas which have been expressed not only in explicit instruction but still more effectively in reaction to our acts." *Human Nature and Conduct* (New York, Henry Holt & Co., 1922), p. 315.

our patient had already socialized his inner conflict. He had identified himself with the army group and he believed in this group and in its ways of looking at things. Their standards were, of course, easier standards, standards which for him represented a concession to his own weaknesses. This being the case, it is obvious that Satan is for him the symbol of the army and its code of sex morality. But his army mates were good fellows after all and he was one of them. Hence his proposed solution. He must try to bring about an understanding between the symbolic representatives of the two groups with which he had been identified. He is to go and see God and get God to come and meet Satan in order that Satan may be converted and bring all his following into the light.

This suggestion is thus not so absurd as at first it seems. It is to be noted that he got well and that he has remained for five years in good condition. He seems really to have succeeded in bringing about some sort of working agreement between the conflicting elements in his personality. It is moreover to be noted that the proposal seems to be rather in line with the teachings of present-day mental hygiene. It is quite likely that our patient's father and his other early guides were over-severe and puritanical in the matter of sex morality. It is hardly to be questioned that organized religion has much to learn about human nature and about the more enlightened ways of managing the powerful sex urge. But the point to which I wish to call particular attention is the fact that to our patient, and likewise to all others who pass through such crisis experiences, *the relationship to the group becomes all important, and that he judges himself by ethical standards which are determined by the group with which he seeks identification and whose approval he needs.* His primary loyalty has been to his parents and the other early guides upon whom he was dependent for support and affection and whose composite impress is represented in his idea of God. Failing to adjust himself to the standards thus set for him he took refuge within a group whose sex code was not determined by the motive of race perpetuation and which therefore dealt leniently with his frailties. The conflict was then revived and precipitated by the experience of fatherhood which brought to the fore the motive of race perpetuation and therefore required reconciliation with that in his social experience which for him represented the abiding and the universal.

In the preceding chapter we have had evidence that our patient is not alone in trying to get God to come and meet Satan. Many are the devices and marvelous the elaborations by which men everywhere seek to avoid condemnation before that inner tribunal known as conscience. To be at one with that which is supreme in our hierarchy of loyalties, that to which men generally give the name of God, is ever essential to mental health; to be isolated or estranged through the consciousness that there is that within which we cannot acknowledge without being condemned means mental disorder and spiritual death. One of the very common methods of avoiding such condemnation is that represented by our patient in his attempt to shift his loyalties. In its extreme form we see this in the delinquent and the criminal, who are at one with themselves but at odds with society. They solve the problem by refusing to recognize their membership in the larger community. Such persons may have been reared in a social environment where it is normal to be delinquent.[5] Commonly, however, their attitude results from rebellion against the primary loyalties and their associated standards. The true delinquent and criminal is characteristically a member of some group. He is, as Dr. Myerson points out, uneasy when he is alone. The thief must belong to some group and have some sense of social support to avoid going insane. There are thus multitudes of men and women who, like our patient, attempt to get rid of the sense of moral failure by identifying themselves with groups which condone or approve the indulgences which they are either unable or unwilling to give up. The average or "normal" man is thus apt to seek the solution of his conflicts by socializing them with a somewhat lowered conscience threshold and comforting himself with the thought that

[5] Clifford Shaw, *The Jack-roller* (Chicago, University of Chicago Press, 1930), chap. 3; also *Delinquency Areas* (Chicago, University of Chicago Press).

he is no worse than his neighbor. And even the church, the institution which seeks to represent that which is permanent and universal in human society, tends constantly to introduce short cuts and protective devices in order to bolster up the moral self-respect of its faulty members. It becomes over-particular about creedal conformity and ritualistic niceties and in other ways it tends to substitute minor for major virtues and loyalties. In trying to get God to come and meet Satan our patient was therefore merely giving expression to the common tendency to seek divine sanction and approval for compromises made in the interests of human frailty. There is thus constant interaction between the needs and frailties of the individual and the ideals and standards of the group. The individual judges himself by the standards of those to whom he gives allegiance and with whom he wishes to be identified, and to be unable to stand before the inner tribunal means for him isolation and destruction. For the sake of his own mental health he must be at one with some group, and his frailties may lead him either to shift his loyalties to a group of easier standards or else to lend his influence to modifying the exacting requirements of the group to which he may belong through birth and early training. The presence of the protective devices with which organized religion is so encumbered means simply that the church is made up in large part of individuals who are trying to serve two masters and are thus not ready to meet the conditions of their fullest self-realization.

The potency of the early influences may be seen in the failure of our patient's attempt to shift his loyalties. To the young child the father, the mother, the early guides, stand as the embodiment of that in the universe upon which he is dependent in a way and to a degree which is never repeated in the course of his development.[6] The impress of their influences, therefore, goes with him through his life and implants in him ideals and standards from which there is no escape except through growth into a larger loyalty and a more

---

[6] The Freudian doctrine that the conscience is the product of the parental influences seems to me frequently to miss the point that the parent is merely the representative of something beyond himself.

comprehensive understanding. Our patient has thus recognized and accepted the parental ideals and standards but he has found difficulty in adjusting himself to them. He has therefore followed the line of least resistance and has sought to escape them by taking refuge in another group. Even though he thus succeeds in finding social support for the indulgence of his unmanageable sex urge, he still feels the superior claim of the parental group and its ideals. He has not grown into a larger loyalty of a more comprehensive understanding. He has merely made a concession to his weaknesses. He is therefore a divided personality.

In such cases Alexander may be right in talking about " an unconscious super-ego " which is distinct from the " conscious conscience " or " ego-ideal." [7] Such a cleavage is however pathological. It is this which constitutes the " divided self," which Professor James has brilliantly described.[8] It is this which made our patient liable to the catastrophe which befell him. He had identified himself with the army group and outwardly accepted its standards without giving up his allegiance to the family group and to the ideals implanted by his early training. The coming of the child, together with the blocking of his vocational self-expression, brought him face to face with the loyalty to which he had been recreant. This meant for him a day of judgment. But no such cleavage should exist in the healthy personality. In any healthy development the primary loyalties and ideals are assimilated and embodied in the expanding organization. There is a constant outreach after the best and the true which results in the outgrowing of the early ideals.

It may be said that the entire social structure, internalized in the form of conscience, is built upon a principle which forbids the disregard or evasion of a primary loyalty but which does permit and, in fact, require that the primary loyalty should be incorporated in a loyalty more comprehensive. According to this view, then, the Freudians are right in insisting upon the im-

[7] *Psychoanalysis of the Total Personality* (Washington, Nervous and Mental Disease Publishing Co., 1930), 20 ff.

[8] *Varieties of Religious Experience* (New York, Longmans, Green and Co., 1902), Lectures VI–VIII.

portance of parental influence in the formation of ideals and standards. Just as truly as the child receives from his parents a physical structure, so also does he take over from his early environment a mental structure which is organized around his primary loyalties. But the ethical ideals and standards which are thus implanted are not fixed and rigid except in pathological cases. Conscience is not just backward-looking. It lies rather, as Professor Hocking contends, on the growing edge of human nature.[9] It represents the awareness of success or failure in maintaining one's status and one's growth. It is the artistic sense which tells us what is or is not fitting in social relationships, long before our clumsy reasons are able to pronounce judgment. And the ideals or standards by which we judge ourselves are determined not so much by the group to which we have belonged, as by that to which we aspire, not so much by the yesterdays as by the tomorrows.

The concern about cosmic affairs and the tendency to personalize the cosmic forces, manifested by our patient, is, as we have seen, characteristic of those disturbances which represent awareness of danger and attempts at reconstruction. It is not characteristic of those cases in which the patient drifts unresistingly down to destruction or in which he attempts to conceal the situation.[10] This is equivalent to saying that in the first type we have religious concern and in the others we do not. We are thus justified in saying that religious concern tends to appear wherever men are facing their difficulties and seeking to become better. The religious attitude is characterized by the outreach after the best and the true and by the attempt to elevate the personal and group loyalties to the level of the cosmic and to make them something more than contemporary and local. Religion is thus social in origin and it seeks to meet the need for social response and security in the attempt to identify the individual self with that which is felt to be universal and abiding in human society. The personalization of this in the idea of God is a consequence not

[9] W. E. Hocking, *Human Nature and Its Re-making* (New Haven, Yale University Press, 1923), pp. 123–4.
[10] Cf. above, pp. 30–43.

merely of the social origin of religion but also of the need of the struggling individual for social support and for relief from the sense of isolation. Because of the social utility and therapeutic value of the belief in a personal God, it seems very doubtful whether a purely humanistic religion can ever make any headway outside of university centers.

In our patient's commission to " get the spirit working " and in his desire to enlist Satan in the task of bringing all men into the light we see an expression of the missionary motive which is commonly characteristic of vital religion. This may be regarded as the reverse side of the motive which prompts the delinquent to seek refuge in a gang. Just as the delinquent seeks social validation for his antisocial tendencies, so the individual who is reaching out for the best seeks to share any new insights which may have come to him and to enlarge their circle of influence. This impulse may be regarded as the root of all organized religion and a necessary consequence of religion's requirement that loyalties should be raised to the cosmic level. Organized religion is thus the attempt to provide for the perpetuation and extension of the profounder insights and the moral achievements of the race and for the co-operative pursuit of the better personal and social life on the basis of an accepted ideal toward which we are moving and of its concomitant hierarchy of values.

We see thus in the case of our patient that the problem of values is very closely associated with the problem of religion. In his religion we see the attempt to raise his loyalties and his value-judgments to the level of the cosmic. In his idea of God we see the symbol with which is associated the thought of those whom he counts most worthy of love and honor. The idea of God thus represents to him that in his social life which he feels to be abiding and universal. It stands to him for that which is supreme in his hierarchy of loyalties. It is the composite image of those whose fellowship and approval he seeks. He therefore judges himself by the standards which are imposed upon him by his religion and associated with his idea of God. Right is that which God approves. Wrong is that which God disapproves. Self-judgment is ever a social judgment [11] and the idea of God is the symbol of the collective at its best.

In thus relating the problem of values to that of religion we are recognizing its personal and subjective nature. Our religion and the ethical ideals and standards which it represents are subject to the accidents of birth and early influences and to personal affinities and choices. But it is also true, as we have said, that religion stands for the earnest outreach after the true and after the best in our social experience. On the basis of clinical observations it can be asserted that no individual is likely to remain permanently satisfied with any loyalty which is for him a lesser one and that protective devices and subterfuges which block growth are seldom if ever effective. Inner unrest and social maladjustment are sure to result. In the fact that there seems thus to be no escape from the primary loyalties and from the ideals and ethical standards which they have inculcated, except through growth into a higher loyalty and a more comprehensive understanding, we may find the basis for an ultimate synthesis of conflicting loyalties and divergent standards. In the enduring and inexorable quest, not of the good — a formula which implies a fixed code and a static morality — but of the best — a formula which implies relativity and calls for continuous growth — we are pointed toward what our patient calls "the millennium, when all men shall be striving together for one goal and for the kingdom of heaven."

It is perhaps not accidental that out of a personal problem with an unmanageable sex drive our patient has been led to concern himself with the problem of world peace. Chance may have had something to do with his enlisting in the army, where he had ample opportunity to become aware of the unhappy state of this sick old world in which "men are always and forever fighting each other." But the problem of loyalties and diverse standards is not without its bearing upon that of war and peace. Conflicting loyalties and diverse standards have in the past been a fruitful

[11] Mead, *Mind, Self, and Society* (Chicago, University of Chicago Press, 1935), p. 255.

source of war and social difficulty, and the tendency toward discord has been greatly accentuated by those who find it much easier to fight for a cause than to live up to their ideals. Many a man who falls far short of his accepted ethical standards and is rather careless about his church attendance will get a glow of righteous satisfaction out of fighting for the Protestant faith in the white nightgown of the K. K. K. Some of the fiercest of wars have been fought in the name of religion, while the superpatriotism so largely responsible for the World War seeks ever to give the finality of religion to its own aims.

This consideration of the case of our peacemaker leads us to the conclusion that the old " good-evil antithesis " is hardly likely ever to become antiquated. Ideas of what is right and wrong may vary from age to age and from one culture to another but the antithesis itself is rooted in the social nature of man and the conditions of social survival and progress. Apart from the social organism man cannot exist. In each individual the organized attitudes of the groups are in some measure internalized. He has some idea of that which the group approves and that which it condemns. According to the scale of values thus determined he judges himself. The presence within himself of anything which he thinks the group would not tolerate will be condemned by himself. It will give rise to a sense of inner disharmony. This, as we have seen, may be dealt with in several ways. The individual may bring himself into harmony with the group by eliminating or else assimilating (socializing) the disturbing elements. He may appeal from his own group and his own primary loyalties to another group. The third alternative is the withdrawal, misinterpretation or progressive disorganization which we see in the various types of mental illness. There is thus no escape from the necessity of passing some sort of moral judgment upon ourselves. The one question is, With which group do we wish to be identified? Whom do we regard supremely worthy of love and honor? The answer to that question will determine the standards of our moral judgment.

The problem of right and wrong thus resolves itself into a question of group attitudes. What we think is right or wrong will be determined by those whose approval we want, and what the group regards as right or wrong will determine its chances of survival in the struggle for existence and the extent to which it will achieve the more abundant life. A boy brought up in the area of family disorganization in a big city may be free from all sense of wrongdoing in the matter of the antisocial acts which his gang approves, but the gang itself has not the capacity for self-perpetuation. It is a parasitic group which has within it the elements of disintegration. It is able to survive only by preying upon an ongoing society. Similarly any religion, any ethical code, any culture, is to be judged by its fruits. Protestant Christianity may thus claim first place among the religions of the world because it is associated with the greatest advancement in science and in social and industrial organization. The Protestant Christian culture has produced the most complex and most highly developed society with the maximum control over the forces of nature. On the other hand, Christendom today is torn with war and hatred between nations and between classes and there is grave danger that it may destroy itself. In the latter case the attitudes and values which it inculcates are likely to perish with it.

If anyone should enter the objection that the problem of values belongs in the field of philosophy rather than in that of science, there is no need to quarrel about words. My point is that values are functions of man's relationship to his environment and ethical values of his relationship to his social environment, particularly to that which he accounts supreme in his hierarchy of loyalties. Such being the case, the problem may be approached empirically on the basis of actual observations and inductive reasoning; and no human behavior is likely to throw more light upon this problem than that of individuals who are grappling with the overwhelming sense of moral failure and isolation and are breaking or broken under the strains of emotional crisis.

VII

THE QUEEN OF THE SCIENCES

Fundamental Postulates of the Humanistic Sciences

Some years ago a study of the Negroes in Chicago was made by a committee of eminent sociologists and social workers. The study grew out of race riots which had disturbed the peace of the community. Its purpose was to get the facts regarding the conditions among thousands of black laborers who had been flocking in from the south. All phases of Negro life were investigated — work, play, housing, family, health, and so forth — in order to provide the basis for intelligent plans to contribute to their welfare and to promote better race relations. In the book that resulted, a book of 670 pages, just four pages were devoted to the Negro's religion and to his church.[1]

This is but one instance of the widespread tendency to neglect the study of religion and religious institutions on the part of those who are charged with the scientific study of human nature, both collective and individual. Few social workers thus give more than passing attention to their clients' philosophy of life. Even in case histories of the mentally ill, the section on religion is commonly dismissed with the statement that the patient is a Protestant or a Catholic. And yet, if our findings are correct, the problem of mental illness centers in the disorganization of the philosophy of life. It has to do with the sufferer's attitude toward his world and his conception of his own place therein. To understand his difficulty without taking account of his religion is therefore an

---

[1] *The Negro in Chicago* (Chicago, University of Chicago Press, 1922).

utter impossibility. And anyone acquainted with Negroes knows how important a part their church plays in their personal and communal life, and how essential it is to take account of their religion in arriving at any true understanding of them.

This tendency to ignore the religious may be seen also in a somewhat scornful attitude toward the professional groups dealing with religion and a tendency to discount their scientific endeavors. In the eyes of our modern intelligentsia no man can be religious and at the same time scientific, for to them the presuppositions of religion and of science are at variance one with the other. Thus it has come to pass that the erstwhile Queen of the Sciences under whose protective care our colleges and even our state universities were founded and nurtured is today a monarch without a throne. The men of today worship at the shrine of science and give to it the same unthinking devotion which formerly was given to the accepted religious dogmas. Meanwhile the term " scientific " has become a sort of shibboleth used commonly with only the haziest conception of its fundamental principles.

In making the attempt to formulate the laws of spiritual life with which theology has to do, as these laws have been revealed through this inquiry, it has seemed proper for me to give a statement of my scientific credo. It may then be clear on what grounds I would claim for theology a place of central importance in that enterprise to which we give the name of science.

In advancing the proposition that theology deserves a place among the sciences, I am assuming with Dewey that science is the co-operative attempt to test and to organize human experience by discovering the constant relationships among changes.[2] Its task, according to Karl Pearson, is the classification of facts and the recognition of their sequence and relative importance.[3] From other forms of reflective thinking, as analyzed by Dewey, it is to be distinguished in that unlike common sense it is not content to stop with the mere coming to mind of practical solutions of a particular difficulty. Neither is it content as in mathematical and philo-

---

[2] *Reconstruction in Philosophy* (New York, Henry Holt & Co., 1920), p. 64.
[3] *Grammar of Science.*

sophical reasoning and untested scientific insight merely to reason out with the aid of memory and imagination the consequences which are involved in the various suggested solutions.[4] Science is the conscious, systematic, co-operative effort to test the various suggested solutions of a difficulty or perplexity by means of empirical observation and experimentation in order to arrive at the universal relationships or laws which may be involved.

I am assuming furthermore that scientific enterprise is based upon certain postulates and follows certain recognized principles. Underlying all its procedures is the assumption that the universe is orderly and subject to the operation of certain laws and that our experience of the external world is trustworthy. The scientist does not, like the acutely disturbed patient and like some philosophers, start out with the assumption that things are not what they seem and then endeavor to get behind experience. He is indeed inclined to be skeptical and hard-headed; he always seeks to look back of appearances and back of the obvious and superficial to underlying causes; he is watchful and critical of the processes of knowing and evaluating experience; but he wastes no time speculating as to whether we can know at all.[5] Neither does he attempt to prove by logical reasoning the existence of an unknowable Absolute. The data of experience he accepts as reliable and explainable in terms of relationships which are universally valid.

The principles of scientific procedure, as nearly as I can analyze them, are as follows:

1. *Empiricism.* The raw material of experience in all its complexity is taken as the starting point. Scientific reasoning is inductive, proceeding from the concrete to the abstract, from the immediate to the remote, from the particular to the general. The scientist does not begin with other men's generalizations and simplifications except as he may apply these to some first-hand observations of his own.

2. *Objectivity.* The personal equation is so far as possible elimi-

[4] E. A. Burt, *Principles and Problems of Right Thinking* (New York, Harper and Bros., 1928), 84 ff.

[5] John Dewey, *Experience and Nature* (Chicago, Open Court Publishing Co., 1926), 19 ff.

nated in that facts and conditions are described so that others can repeat the experiment or observe for themselves and draw their own independent conclusions.

3. *Continuity.* New phenomena are explained in terms of previous observation and generalization. The unknown must be related to the known.

4. *Particularity.* The field of inquiry must be limited and the problem clearly defined. It is necessary to devote oneself to some small portion of the universe and for the time being neglect the rest.

5. *Universality.* The particular can be understood only in the light of the general and the aim of all scientific endeavor is to discover relationships that are universally valid.

6. *Economy.* In the words of the old scholastic law, " Neither more nor more onerous causes must be assumed than are necessary to account for the phenomena." From this principle follow two important corollaries:

(a) Between two theories, each of which accounts for a certain set of facts, that one is to be accepted which brings them into unity with other fields of experience.

(b) The scale of accuracy of any piece of investigation must be exactly suited to the end in view and to the character of the material under investigation. It may be as much an error to use too fine a scale of accuracy as one that is too rough.

7. *Disinterestedness.* The desire to find the truth must be supreme. Rigid honesty and accuracy and the ability to understand and discount personal bias must characterize the good scientific worker.

In adopting these principles I would however make certain explanations and reservations.

By " empiricism " I do not mean that one must begin with the data of experience without an intelligent idea of what he ought to look for or that the data of experience must be limited to sense perceptions. The ideas of my patients, even though elusive, are just as properly objects of empirical investigation as their pulse rate or their blood pressure. And any definite utterances of theirs are much more direct and objective indications of what is going on in their minds than any mere descriptions of their behavior. In this inquiry I have begun with certain definite leads drawn from my own experience and I have sought by statistical methods to verify or disprove these hypotheses. My own experience has however been excluded from the field of inquiry. Even though I look upon myself as one who has visited a far-off country and even though my report is adequately documented and carefully worked out, I cannot help being a bit sensitive about subjecting it to that general scrutiny which scientific objectivity requires. What I have tried to do in this inquiry and what seems to me central in the principle of empiricism is to deal at first hand with the raw material of some definite segment of human life. And just as no historian worthy of the name is content to accept on authority the simplified statement of some other historian regarding the problem under investigation, so I have sought to begin not with the ready-made formulations contained in books but with the living human documents and with actual social conditions in all their complexity.

I would also make it clear that by " continuity " I do not mean scientific determinism. I am ready to agree that no explanation must be permitted except in terms of tested and ordered experience and that the scientific worker must be held to his task of discovering relationships. But a methodological principle must not be confused with a philosophical proposition. The excellent purpose of trying to explain the human mind in terms of objective behavior becomes at once an absurdity when it is carried over into the proposition that there is no such thing as consciousness and that thought is nothing but implicit vocalization. So also the insistence upon explaining the unknown in terms of the known is something very different from the proposition that there can be nothing new or creative in human experience. The historian is thus right in seeking to relate Jesus' idea of the Kingdom of God and of his own messiahship to ideas current among the Jews of his time. He is also right in pointing out that the identification of Jesus with God, such as we find in the letter to the

Colossians, resembles ideas characteristic of the eastern mystery religions and that it is not found in those Jewish documents of that period which have been preserved to us. But when the historian goes on to assert that Jesus' idea of the Kingdom and of his own rôle in that Kingdom could have been derived *only* from the stream of tradition and that the letter to the Colossians could not have been written by a Jew and therefore not by Paul, I take the liberty of being skeptical.

The years which I spent in the study of the social and religious conditions in rural Missouri and Tennessee and Kansas revealed to me many ideas and customs current there of which I had heard nothing in the rarefied atmosphere of the theological school from which I had just come. I am very sure that if a similar survey could have been made in Palestine in the first century it would have brought to light many streams of Jewish thinking of which we know nothing today. We must not forget that what has been preserved to us is the result of a highly selective process and is even then very fragmentary. Our present knowledge of Jewish life and thought in that period is thus highly oversimplified. My skepticism regarding the necessity of limiting the ideas of Jesus or of Paul to what we know of the stream of tradition in their time is all the greater because of my observations in the mental hospital. These furnish abundant evidence that in the searching experiences of human life there is a tendency to disregard the ideas and culture patterns of the particular age and race and to produce spontaneously just such formulations as we see in Jesus and in Paul.[6] These crisis experiences tend also to produce combinations so new as to be new creations. According to the law of economy these observations of human nature under stress offer a simpler explanation of Jesus' idea of the Kingdom and of his own messiahship than that based on our fragmentary records of what Palestinian Jews were thinking in the first century. They also indicate that for any man who felt, as Paul did, that the heavens had been opened to him and that the risen Jesus had ap-

---

[6] See pp. 134–35; also John Dollard, " The Psychotic Person Seen Culturally," *American Journal of Sociology*, March, 1934.

peared and spoken to him, nothing would have been more probable than that he would associate that appearance of Jesus with his idea of God. It would be quite unnecessary to assume that he must have been influenced by the mystery religions, for our observations of what men think in times of crisis and upheaval brings these facts into unity with a wider and more readily verifiable field of experience. These observations also furnish evidence of spontaneous and creative elements in human nature, which may influence the stream of tradition quite as much as the stream of tradition may account for them.

I am also skeptical regarding " scientific disinterestedness " and I have used that term only because it is widely current. Loyalty to the truth at whatever cost must indeed be the ideal of the scientist, but that does not mean that he must be just a detached observer. Such a thing would be neither possible nor desirable. The often-repeated assertion that the scientist must have no preconceptions regarding his data seems to me plain nonsense. A student of the New Testament times must indeed saturate himself in the life and thought of that period as revealed through the existing documents in the effort to discover its distinguishing characteristics, but to say, as some do say, that he should approach his sources without any preconceptions regarding human nature is a bit naïve. The result could hardly fail to be an uncritical projection of his own personal experiences upon those sources. His only safeguard is to become clearly conscious of what he is doing and to bring to bear upon the sources a better understanding of the enduring elements in human nature. It should moreover be clearly recognized that it is only the existence of preconceptions which makes scientific work possible. The expert is the man whose previous experience enables him to know what to look for. To ask the right question and to have a really fruitful lead is the basis of all worth-while contributions to science. Such leads are the working hypotheses of the scientist, which he seeks to prove or disprove, and even though he may start with a multiplicity of hypotheses, once he begins to formulate his conclusions the chosen hypothesis is apt to become for him a veritable vested interest. After his system is well worked out, it may be as hard to modify as the delusional system of the paranoic. Only the exceptional scientist is able to attain in any measure to the ideal of open-mindedness and honesty. Certainly the recent war did not furnish us with any great demonstration of scientific disinterestedness. In fact our great universities on both sides were hotbeds of the war spirit with all its bitterness and unhappy distortion of facts. Scientists, after all, are human and all that we can expect of them is that they should be able to reserve judgment when the evidence is not all in, and ready to modify their conclusions in the light of new evidence.

A note is also needed regarding the principles of " particularity and universality." The scientist must indeed devote himself to some small portion of the universe and for the time being neglect the rest. The necessity of choosing a clearly defined problem and of limiting the field of inquiry is a lesson the beginner often has difficulty in learning. He is apt to want to study the reconciliation of nations rather than the forces at work in some neighborhood gang or the habits of algae in some little pool. But it is equally true that his ability to discover the universal laws that are operative in the neighborhood gang or in the pool of algae is going to depend upon the comprehensiveness and justice of the understanding that he is able to bring to bear upon his own particular task. Narrow specialization may chance upon findings of real importance, but it also results in much unintelligent and unfruitful fact-finding such as has cluttered up our scientific periodicals during these years of mushroom growth in our colleges. A balance must always be maintained between the two. There can be no great scientist who is not master of some special field and who is not able also to see his particular specialty in its general perspective. In the present inquiry I have, in accordance with the principle of particularity, disregarded the organic and structural factors in the behavior of my patients, except to note the inconclusive results of physiological studies in the research cases. Whatever may be the truth of the commonly accepted view that mind and body are one, I see nothing to be gained from any attempt on my part to give explanations in terms of stimulus-response mechanisms or of the autonomic functions of the personality. Even though I were an expert in both psychology and physiology, the first step would seem to be the relatively simple task of determining the relationships within different orders of events, before attempting the more complicated and baffling problem of the correlation between the mental and the physical. I have therefore given my explanations in terms of desires and emotions and social relationships. I trust, however, that I have not failed to see my own contribution in its general setting nor to give due respect to the contributions of other workers.

The application of these principles to the study of human nature has been beset with very great difficulties. The extreme complexity of human nature makes controlled experimentation of very limited applicability, and representatives of the exact sciences have not been sparing in their criticisms. The tendency in the era just closing has been to meet these criticisms by trying to fulfill the conditions of exactness and of experimental control called for by the older sciences. Sociologists have thus gone in for statistics, often forgetting that statistics are useful only in verifying hypotheses gained through the study of particular cases and situations. Sometimes they have attempted the wholesale application of such methods to unreliable data. Psychologists have retired into their laboratories to busy themselves with elaborate apparatus for the controlled study of stimulus-response mechanisms, to the neglect of the great driving forces of human life, love and hate and fear and anger. They have gone in for ambitious attempts to measure intelligence and even character, forgetting the fact that averages apply only to averages and are of very limited value in sizing up a particular individual. At the very time that physicists have been giving up the old ideas regarding the conservation of energy and the immutability of natural law, we see humanistic workers stressing scientific determinism. They have also accepted the dictum that science is not concerned with purposes and values and some have even gone to the absurd length of denying the reality of consciousness. The humanistic scientists, in brief, in their efforts to take over the methodology of the exact sciences have violated one of the cardinal principles of scientific procedure. They have been making use of a scale of accuracy that is not warranted by the material with which they are dealing nor by the kind of yardsticks at their disposal. They are like surveyors whose assignment calls for the use of compass and pacing, but who give their measurements in tenths of inches. And meantime, all too often, they lose sight of that which is distinctive in human nature.

In recent years a new point of view has been introduced chiefly through insights gained in the study of the mentally ill. In recognizing that mental disorder is best explained in terms of the reaction of the individual to his environment, a new emphasis has been placed upon the need of considering the organism as a whole. There is a growing recognition that the whole is something vastly more than an aggregation of parts and that its reactions cannot be explained as some simple functions of the laws of the independent parts.[7] The organism as a whole has desires and purposes, it recognizes some scale of values and its desires must be organized around a plan much as bodily organs are. More and more the psychiatrist has come to see that he is dealing with the results of mankind's experimentation with emotions. He is coming to see that ideas and emotions are to his patients tremendous realities and only as they are taken into account will it be possible to understand their difficulties. The new emphasis upon the wishes in the study of human nature has probably been the great contribution of Freudian psychology. Freud himself, together with his more orthodox followers, might not agree with this. He has given his explanations rather in terms of past causes and he has sought to keep his psychology within a deterministic framework. But his findings point distinctly toward a psychology that is dynamic and purposive. This inquiry aligns itself with Jung in holding that the yesterdays are important only in so far as they throw light upon the tomorrows, and that to understand men either individually or collectively one must first of all ask what they want and what they are trying to do. Past history and causation must certainly

[7] A. D. Ritchie, *Scientific Method* (New York, Harcourt, Brace & Co., 1921), p. 179.

not be neglected, but to give explanations in terms of purposes and values and to recognize that the organism as a whole has at least some limited power of choice would thus be of the very essence of the humanistic sciences.

This new emphasis upon the organism as a whole and its reaction to the total environment, together with the recognition of desire and purpose and the reality of choice in the attempt to understand human nature, leads at once to the dethroned Queen of the Sciences. For theology has always been concerned with the motivating beliefs of men regarding their origin and destiny and their relationship to the universe. It has dealt with that which is supreme in the hierarchy of desires and values and with the choices which favor or impede maximum self-realization.

In thus recognizing theology as a proper field of scientific investigation, we are concerned with its subject matter, not with its traditional methodology. I do not propose to begin with any abstract formulations concerning the existence and nature of God, the depravity of man, and the plan of salvation as these doctrines have been handed down in organized Christianity. Our task in the present chapter will be to review the material presented in the preceding chapters in the light of the problems with which theology is concerned. Our generalizations will thus be based upon the empirical study of a limited number of persons, most of whom have passed through periods of crisis and mutation with radical changes in personality, some for the better, some for the worse. Examining the beliefs of these individuals, each in its own context amid the complex entanglements of actual life, and taking account of the consequences which have followed from particular choices and reaction patterns, we may be able to arrive at some valid generalizations regarding the meaning of the idea of God, the nature and function of religion, and the conditions under which maximum self-realization is likely to be achieved.

In choosing for study those who have passed through crisis experiences, we have a definite reason. The normal or average man does not as a rule concern himself to any great extent about his relationship to the universe. He is usually engrossed in his immediate pursuits, and in so far as he occupies himself with the problems relating to his ultimate destiny, his thinking is generally along traditional and conventional lines. But in times of crisis and extremity the individual is usually absorbed in the problems of why he is in the world and of his relationship to the forces upon which he feels himself dependent. He is face to face with the issues of life and death, of success and failure, from the standpoint of the abiding values. He feels himself in direct contact with the unseen and mysterious forces of the universe, some friendly and some unfriendly. He finds himself cut loose from the culture patterns of his particular race and time and shoved forth into the timeless and limitless unknown. Out of such profound experiences there are those who emerge with new insights to become poets, philosophers, prophets, molders of the traditions which the masses accept. The characteristic ideation of primitive peoples, which, as has been frequently pointed out, bears many points of resemblance to psychotic thinking, is due probably in large part to their much greater readiness to accept without discrimination the reports of those who pass through such searching experiences. With the advance of culture and enlightenment our ideas concerning man's place in the universe are determined more and more by a growing knowledge of the age of the earth, of the process of evolution, of the movements of the stars, and the like. Nevertheless a critical study of the inner world of thought and feeling and volition, as it is revealed to us in the great crisis experiences, when the results, for better or for worse, of the individual's experiments with life are being unfolded, may also contribute something to our understanding of man's nature and destiny.

Man and His Destiny

From this study of individuals who pass through periods of emotional crisis and mutation several things stand out in clear relief:

1. Most persons in these periods of crisis feel that their eyes have been opened to unsuspected meanings and possibilities in their lives. The so-called " normal " range of vision becomes for them inadequate and superficial. They look upon it as character-

ized by an absorption in trivialities and a yielding to the unacceptable, when all the time issues of infinite importance were at stake both for themselves and for others. Of our 173 hospital cases, 57 thought some sort of world change was impending and 53 thought of themselves as having therein a rôle of cosmic significance. These ideas were found to be characteristic of panic reactions and attempts at reconstruction as contrasted with the malignant reactions of drifting and concealment. Various symbols were used but the fundamental idea was the same. The individual felt within himself, at least in retrospect, unsuspected and infinite possibilities.

Equally common were ideas of death and nullity. There was in many cases an overwhelming sense of worthlessness and infinitesimal smallness. Not infrequently the two ideas occurred in conjunction. The man who identified himself with God was quite likely to think of himself as a zero quantity.

About 15 of our group of patients had ideas of previous incarnation. Their eyes had been opened so that they could see back to the beginning of all creation. They had been first one and then another historic character. Some even thought of themselves as passing through the various stages of animal evolution. Several thought they were journeying all around the universe, visiting Mars and Saturn and the moon and even taking a little jaunt to Arcturus.

2. Corresponding somewhat to the old ideas of total depravity we see in these persons a great reservoir of unacceptable instinctual cravings which have been standing in the way of higher potentialities and all too often engulf and destroy them. Radical evil is a terrific reality and the fears we see in the disturbed patient are not without foundation. There *is* such a thing as disintegration or damnation and no philosophy of life which fails to take account of that is really facing the facts. It is moreover to be noted that the patient who is alive to his danger and recognizes it for the grim reality that it is has the best chance of making a good recovery.

3. " As a man thinketh in his heart, so is he," is a principle which stands out in clear relief. The mentally ill are for the most part

those who are living in the realm where ideas have the value of reality. To the mentally ill the presence of an unacceptable thought or craving is just as terrible as the actual committing of some forbidden act. Mental disorder seems thus primarily a matter of emotion and volition, of attitude and belief. Above all it arises out of a failure to organize these into a philosophy of life which will enable the individual to assimilate his new experiences and make decisions as to what to do in a given situation. Central in such an organization is some conception of the self and of its place in the universe, some conception of the rôle one is to fill and of the scale of values by which success or failure is to be judged. This organization of experience is infinitely delicate and complex. If we speak of this as the " philosophy of life " it must be understood that it includes not only the intellectual but also the emotional and volitional, not only that which is in the focus of attention, but the vast background of previous experience, possibly racial as well as individual. According to Dewey all these are present and to some extent operative even in the simplest act or thought.[8]

4. Concerning the possibility of the survival of the personality after death this inquiry provides no basis for an answer. From the standpoint of empirical observation all we can say is, When a man is dead he stays dead. Neither have we any new light upon the relationship of body and mind. The painstaking and elaborate physiological research work done on the hospital cases which we have studied failed, as we have seen, to reveal any organic disease as characteristic either of schizophrenia or of its several types. The general tendency today seems to be away from the sweeping claims formerly made regarding the physical basis of the personality. The extreme theories regarding the localization of brain functions, which prevailed thirty years ago, have now been swept away along with phrenology. The more recent studies indicate that the brain tends to function as a whole and that destruction of brain tissue, so far as the intellectual processes are concerned, tends to cause general impairment of function rather than destruction of specific

[8] *Experience and Nature* (Chicago, Open Court Publishing Co., 1926), 299 ff.

functions.[9] It also remains true, as Bergson pointed out years ago, that no one has ever succeeded in localizing memory. In the aphasias there is a tendency to forget in a certain order, first proper nouns, then common nouns, then adjectives and last of all verbs. There is also in the aphasias an ability to recall under the influence of strong emotion. Bergson concludes that such facts as these indicate that the brain is merely an instrument through which something else functions which may be quite independent of the mere physical organism.[10]

The investigations of psychic phenomena have of course been equally unavailing in the production of proof of survival. Undoubtedly many individuals have found what for them is proof, but it has remained impossible to fulfill the conditions of objective demonstration. Experiences of communication with a spiritual world remain personal and private and cannot be repeated under conditions that will be convincing to others.

The question of survival after death is thus still an open one. There is no compelling evidence either for or against belief in survival. It must be left to each man to follow in this matter the implications of his general philosophy of life. This inquiry does reveal however that those who in great crises of life have stood on the threshold of the unknown all agree in feeling themselves continuous with something beyond, something that has been before this present life and something that will continue to be. It may also be pointed out that the ideas of these persons regarding their relationship to the universe are not far out of accord with what our growing knowledge of the external world is revealing to us regarding man's infinite complexity and his infinitesimal littleness.

THE IDEA OF GOD

The idea of God was much in evidence in all of our acutely disturbed patients as one element of their characteristic religious

---

[9] Karl Lashley, *Brain Mechanisms and Intelligence* (Chicago, University of Chicago Press, 1929). See also Pierre Marie, " Existe-t-il chez l'Homme, des Centres Préformés ou Innés du Langage? " *Questions Neurologiques d'Actualité* (Paris, Masson & Cie, 1922).

[10] Henri Bergson, *L'Energie Spirituelle* (Paris, F. Alcan, 1922), pp. 53–61.

concern. This idea cropped out even in those who had not previously been religiously inclined, as a manifestation of the tendency to personalize that upon which in time of crisis one feels dependent. Some of our patients in the period of disturbance even went to the point of personalizing the sun and the moon and the stars.

The orthodox Freudian interpretation of this tendency toward personalization would be in terms of regression to an infantile stage of development. A better explanation would seem to be that it stands for the fundamental human need of love and of racial solidarity. Whatever the metaphysical reality back of the idea of God, that idea represents to the individual who uses the term the composite impress of those with whom he seeks identification, those whose love is necessary to him, and who stand supreme in his hierarchy of loyalties.

Evidence of the social nature of man we have found in the fact that the primary evil in functional mental illness is to be found in the sense of moral failure and isolation. We have thus seen that the assimilation of new experience is coincidental with socialization. We assimilate the new experience by bringing it into conscious relationship with the framework of social experience as accepted by our chosen group. Any new experience which cannot be so related, in so far as it is significant, remains a source of trouble as potent as unassimilated food. To have that in one's life which one is afraid to tell for fear of condemnation by those who are accounted worthy of love and honor is isolation, and isolation means death. This means that no matter whether a man be consciously religious or not, there is deep in his heart the need of being at one with those whom he loves and to whom he owes allegiance. The idea of God is to be regarded as a symbol of that need and of that allegiance. It stands for that which is regarded as enduring and universal in the society to which we belong and of which we feel ourselves a part.

The fact that in so many of our cases sexual maladjustment looms very large leads to a further suggestion. It should be recognized that the problem of sex derives its significance from the fact that here one is dealing with that which is vital to the ongoing process of race perpetuation and improvement. For this the individual exists. All civilization is founded upon the readiness of the individual to give his life for his family, his tribe, his nation. Not a child comes into the world but some woman has to go down to the gates of death to make it possible and in time of danger and of war what is expected from all is too fresh in our memories to need more than mention. The idea of God serves as the symbol of racial solidarity. It stands for that for which we must be ready to give our lives if the race is not to disintegrate and perish. It represents the assertion of religious faith that the structure of society is based on love and that even in giving our lives we find them again.

This inquiry has not revealed any evidence which would indicate that the idea of God as exemplified either in the hospital patients or in the men of religious genius whom we have studied included any particular view regarding his nature or attitude to the universe or to inorganic nature. The idea of God as an omnipotent creator is by no means characteristic. In the men of religious genius the tendency is rather to think of God as a friend and guide. Many of our patients, together with some who are not patients, " get chummy with God." They bring him down to their own level and, as we have seen, they tend to identify themselves with him. In not a few cases they fear for him. God himself is in danger. He is beset by enemies or he is blocked or thwarted in his purposes. Some even think of him as dead. The general tendency in the deep psychoses is a reversion to a rather primitive form of animism in which life and intelligence are attributed even to inanimate objects, and mystery and hidden meanings are everywhere.

Several explanations of these ideas so common in the acute disturbances present themselves for consideration. The first is suggested by the common coexistence of the ideas of world catastrophe and of the exalted rôle which the patient himself is to play in that catastrophe. The idea of world catastrophe, as we have seen,[11] is best explained as a projection of the inner catastrophe. It repre-

[11] See pp. 103–4; also 138–39.

sents the fact that the patient has become completely absorbed in his own personal fate and that in his own inner world the self is or should be monarch. That there is an identification with God or with Christ is therefore not to be wondered at. It is due precisely to the fact that the individual is living inside his own personal inner world, where he himself should rule. That he should think of God as in danger or subject to the attacks of enemies or limited and thwarted, or that he should feel himself surrounded by all sorts of fantastic and fearsome beings, follows inevitably from the personal situation which is being projected.

Another explanation which by no means conflicts with this one is Jung's hypothesis of a racial or collective unconscious.[12] Just as our bodies represent the corporealized experience of countless generations, so also each individual has within him a vast reservoir of racial memories, not yet fixed in organic patterns but capable of being revivified, especially in time of emotional turmoil when the profounder levels of the mental life are stirred. The idea of God would thus be one of these racial memories or " archetypes " — something implanted in human nature and sure to crop out in time of stress and danger. This theory of the racial unconscious has received no widespread acceptance in the psychiatric world. It does however offer a means of bringing order into what is otherwise a confused mass of facts and in so far as it accomplishes this it is worthy of credence. It is moreover to be noted that it has not a little in common with religious insight at its best. It is particularly to be compared with the idea of the indwelling Holy Spirit, of the immanence of God, and with Emerson's idea of the Oversoul.

From the standpoint of this inquiry we may note that the idea of God is not without therapeutic significance.

It stands first of all for a unifying principle in both the individual and social philosophy of life. I was forcibly struck by this fact some years ago in connection with a study of the therapeutic influence of spiritualism in connection with a case on which I was working. I visited eight different mediums whose names and

---

[12] *Two Essays on Analytical Psychology;* see also p. 107.

addresses and hours of meeting had been given me by my patient. The outstanding impression left upon me was the disorganizing influence of their séances. Each medium assumed that he was under the control of some particular discarnate spirit, in each case a different one, and whenever he gave a message, that message purported to come from other discarnate spirits whom he saw hovering about the head of the person for whom it was intended. The whole thing was conducted in an atmosphere which was pervaded with the sense of the uncanny and mysterious. What struck me was the inevitable tendency of such performances to make for a disorganized universe. These discarnate spirits were nothing more than a conglomerate horde of supernatural beings of a low ethical order, some of them being distinctly diabolical. I was not surprised to find that the mediums themselves all recognized the danger, especially to the beginner, of " sitting in the silence." In the churches on the other hand, even in the Holy Roller missions, the attention was centered upon the one God, whose great concern it was that his children should live righteous and holy lives. This idea of God thus has a unifying effect not only upon the individual but upon the group in that it provides all with a common object of loyalty and makes for an organized universe. It thus tends also to develop those common standards and ways of looking at things which result from a common " super-ego." This according to Freud is the basis of any particular culture.

I was also struck in these same Holy Roller missions with the social significance of their idea of God. He was for them one who understands, one to whom they could go with all their problems and difficulties with the assurance that he would not turn them away. In a number of conversion experiences which were reported to me it seemed clear that what had happened was a reorganization with unification and socialization beginning at the very core of the being. This seems to be clearly the intent of the acute upheavals which we find in the hospital and what has actually happened in the case of such men as George Fox. The individual who has shared in that experience has found what for him is the most important thing in the world, something which dwarfs all else into insignificance and enables him, if need be, to stand alone against all contemporary society. In more than one of my patients who have passed through that experience and have reorganized their lives on that basis, I have seen striking examples of an indomitable courage and faith and fortitude in the face of discouragement and misunderstanding which are truly comparable to the spirit manifested by Jeremiah and Fox. That experience gave them faith to attempt the impossible and it kept them steady and unembittered even when they met with nothing but frustration.

With such courage and faith and loyalty, why these prophets on our hospital wards did not attain to something of greater value is a question which suggests a further consideration of no little importance. Their fatal mistake, as I see it, has lain in the failure to recognize and heed that old injunction of true religious insight which requires that we should walk humbly with God. This my hospital prophets had failed to do. They had brought the divine down to their own level. They had indeed found inner unification and they succeeded in maintaining it against great odds but only at very great cost. Their universe had become no bigger than themselves. They had not learned with Paul to think of the divine as something that lived within them as a future possibility to be achieved at the cost of sacrifice and struggle. It was for them something already attained. In dealing with such persons I never try to shake their faith in themselves or in the value of their experience. I try rather to help them to take the next step of freeing the divine from their idea of themselves so as to make possible a larger universe.

The requirement of humility and reverence may, I think, be regarded as basic in the religious attitude. It is a requirement which applies equally well to the religious crank and zealot and to the cocksure person who may call himself a scientist but who has no respect for the beliefs of others and no understanding of the beauty and magnitude and mystery of the universe and of his own small place therein. He also, as Jung suggests, has become a God in his own eyes. The man without humility and without reverence is out of right relationship with the universe and with the society of which he is a part. With the attitude of reverence it makes no great difference what particular religious formulation one may or may not use — the values involved in religious belief are retained.

SIN AND SALVATION

Our inquiry has revealed two major groups of " sinners," those who are at odds with society and those who are at odds with themselves. The first group in their extreme forms we find in our jails and reform schools. They are those who have rejected loyalty to parents and to organized society and are comfortable about it. Forming groups of their own and supporting each other in their antisocial attitudes, they may even take pride in their lawbreaking escapades. The other group we find in our mental hospitals. They are those who accept the primary loyalties but have failed to measure up to the standards which they feel to be required of them. They are well-meaning and they want to do right but they stand condemned in their own eyes. There is that in their lives which they are afraid to tell for fear of condemnation. They have not been able to pay the price of growth by renouncing desires and tendencies which belong to an earlier stage of development.

It is with the latter group that our inquiry has been mainly concerned. Among them we have found three chief groups. There are in the first place those who make no attempt to face their problems. They merely follow the line of least resistance, allowing their difficulties to accumulate. This course tends toward disintegration and destruction. The second group is composed of those who have resorted to some of the many concealment devices in order to preserve their self-esteem and escape the sense of personal failure. Among these devices we have recognized the substitution of minor for major virtues and loyalties, escape into activity and self-assertion, delusional misinterpretation, shifting of responsibility upon other persons or objects, and the taking refuge in illness. We have found that the end result of such methods was arrested development. The unsolved problems were likely to become the source of all sorts of pathological symptoms through which stabilization on an unsatisfactory basis is maintained. Such persons do not often get well, neither do they often go all to pieces. Finally we have found those who in attempting to face their difficulties become much disturbed. Among these there were not a few who recovered. There were also many who went hopelessly to pieces. We concluded therefore that such disturbances were not in themselves evils but were rather analogous to fever or inflammation in the physical organism. They were attempts at cure or reconstruction, which tended to make or break.

Any contribution which this inquiry may be able to make to this problem of sin and salvation must be based chiefly upon what we have discovered regarding the meaning of these acute disturbances.

In the psychopathological approach to the problem of sin and salvation (mental illness and its cure) most of what has been written has come from those who deal with psychoneurotic disorders. Some of these have a great deal to say about ceremonialism. Reik finds this in psychoneuroses to be a means of bringing about a certain equilibrium and allowing the forbidden tendencies to get by.[13] Others, notably Alexander, dealing with the same phenomena find a more inclusive formula in the " need for punishment." He regards self-punishment in its various manifestations as the " counterfeit coinage " by which the unacceptable cravings are permitted to buy indulgence. Every neurosis he explains as an attempt to cling to an instinctual satisfaction which has been condemned by conscience. This comes about through the axiomatic assumption that by means of punishment and suffering one achieves not only absolution from sin but a justification for committing it.[14] This assumption, he holds, is the foundation of all primitive religious systems in which sacrifice serves to appease an avenging deity. Its origin he finds in the fact that from early

[13] Theodor Reik, *Psychoanalytic Studies of Ritual* (New York, Norton and Co., 1934).

[14] Franz Alexander, *Psychoanalysis of the Total Personality* (Washington, Nervous and Mental Disease Publishing Co., 1930), p. 94.

childhood instinct gratification and punishment have been associated. The child has learned moreover that following punishment he may expect a renewal of affection from his parents. He
may also have found that if he beats them to it and punishes himself he may escape punishment at their hands. The adult who
blames himself and punishes himself may thus be seeking to buy
the leniency of his " super-ego " at the same time that he clings to
the gratification he is unable to renounce. In the obsessional or
compulsion neuroses we have a type of solution in which the individual by means of his symptoms is able at the same time to appease both masters, conscience and instinct. In this way a certain
equilibrium is brought about and tension and anxiety are allayed.
In manic-depressive disorders Alexander sees a solution in which
the claims of conscience and those of instinct are satisfied in successive periods. First one and then the other is in the ascendant.
The presence of anxiety and panic means that no equilibrium has
as yet been attained.

These views are in line with our findings. We would however
place such solutions among the malignant concealment reactions
and contrast them sharply with the acute panic and upheaval.
The meaning of the latter, at least in the more hopeful cases, is to
be found not in any attempt to let unacceptable cravings get by.
It is rather an attempt to eliminate them and thus bring about a
unification on the basis of accepted ideals and purposes. The
ideal self, the super-ego, or whatever name one may prefer to use,
thus becomes the new center of the personality. Hence the ideas
of cosmic identification which occur so frequently in such reactions. It is true that the attempt is not generally successful and
that following the period of panic and severity the unacceptable
tendencies are apt to assert themselves again. Nevertheless in
certain men of unquestioned religious genius, such as George
Fox and Emanuel Swedenborg and Saul of Tarsus, we have instances in which the individual passes triumphantly through the
period of acute conflict and succeeds in bringing about a successful
reorganization on the basis of his highest loyalties. We have been
led further to the conclusion that these profound disturbances and

upheavals of the personality bear a close relationship to the eruptive type of happy solutions of inner conflicts which Starbuck has described in his study of the religious conversion experience. They are also closely related to the mystical experiences in general which have figured so prominently in the history of religion. They are thus problem-solving experiences, attempts at reorganization, which call forth hidden sources of power and under favorable conditions do succeed in bringing about a progressive socialization and unification of the personality.

The acute disturbance, together with the religious conversion experience to which it is so closely related, thus stands for complete commitment to that which is supreme in the individual's hierarchy of loyalties. It is the desperate attempt in the face of an accumulation of difficulties to get rid of all that is alien to our accepted ideals and to bring about the needed rebirth or reorganization. From this standpoint the ideas of death and rebirth which recur so frequently in acute disturbances are by no means accidental. They represent the exact meaning of the experience.

In the light of this interpretation we may be inclined to regard neurotic self-punishment from a somewhat different standpoint than that of the psychoanalysts. In many cases, at least, instead of being a means of evasion it may be an attempt at self-discipline. It may thus represent the desperate striving for self-control. And even in those cases in which the psychoanalyst is correct in regarding it as a means of evasion, it may derive its effectiveness not so much from the more or less fortuitous association of punishment and relief but from the more fundamental principle that it looks toward that complete commitment and devotion without which the pearl of great price is not to be had. It stands thus for a true objective. The difficulty is that most mental sufferers have not been able to pay the price and go through with the task they have undertaken.

This requirement of complete commitment even to the point of self-sacrifice is seen in the Christian doctrine of the cross. It is however a sad reflection upon frail human nature that Jesus' own teaching regarding the significance of his death has been so strangely misconstrued. If we can trust gospel accounts, Jesus proclaimed repeatedly in words whose meaning seems perfectly clear that his course was an example and a challenge to his followers and that no man could be his disciple unless he was willing to give up all that he had and follow him. And yet this doctrine of the cross has become the historic doctrine of the vicarious atonement, according to which, as it is commonly interpreted, Jesus gave his life to satisfy the demands of justice and thereby paid the price which enables those who believe in him to obtain salvation in a life hereafter. Jesus' commanding challenge has thus all too often become just another means of evasion.

Some light upon this strange transformation of Jesus' teaching may be gained by a consideration of the situation as regards criminal law. Even today in enlightened America our criminal law is still based upon the old principle of " an eye for an eye and a tooth for a tooth." It is a system for dealing out retribution. When a man does something wrong the punishment is made to fit the crime. If he attacks another man and that man dies, he may be sent to the electric chair. If the other man is merely injured, the severity of the punishment will be determined by the seriousness of the injury. Criminal law takes little account of motive. It still looks upon the crime rather than the criminal. It is based upon fear and upon vengeance. And this attitude which we find in America today is the attitude which we find the world over, not only today but back through the centuries. It is the common way in all times and among all races of enforcing the " thou-shalt-nots." All too often it is also the method used to enforce discipline in the home.

Now the death of Jesus seems to have stood in his own mind for another principle. It was for him the last full measure of devotion to the Love which he believed to rule the universe. It was the bold declaration of his faith that self-realization does not come merely to the victorious survivors but also to those who give their lives for the group. It was the bold declaration of the principle that the redemption of the many is brought about through the sacrificial devotion of the few and it summoned men to enlist in that sacrificial task. It was his proclamation of the good news that in such devotion rather than in conventional morality and success lies the way of salvation. It thus represented the same discovery that Paul made in his doctrine of the spirit as opposed to the law. It was a shift from a static to a dynamic morality which found the good life not in outward correctness but in self-forgetful devotion to the best and brought to the man overwhelmed by his sins the offer of a new chance. It gave the assurance that Love is in control, a Love that looks upon the heart and honors a man not so much for what he has already attained but for what he is in process of becoming.

Such a doctrine is truly good news to those who have a genuine hunger and thirst after the better life and who feel their own need. But of those who have made up the Christian church the great majority have had no enkindling vision. Their membership in the church has been determined chiefly by the fact that they have been born into it and they have wanted to maintain their loyalty to their parents and their parents' God on the easiest possible terms. Hence the doctrine of the vicarious atonement as it has been so generally interpreted. Now this doctrine has not been without religious value even in its popular form. It has enabled multitudes of people to believe that Love is in control in the universe and it has brought to them peace and comfort. But it is obvious that the complacent acceptance of the sacrifice of others is something wholly different from the recognition of the challenge which the death of Jesus brings to us to follow in his footsteps and to give ourselves to a life of self-forgetful devotion and adventurous con-secration to the cause for which he gave his life. The doctrine of the cross has thus all too often been twisted into just another means of evading the inexorable requirement of complete commitment to the task of bringing in the world that ought to be. And so our criminal law is still based upon retribution and fear, and hatred and cutthroat competition still hold sway in a civilization that calls itself Christian.

In addition to those who attempt to maintain their loyalty by paying counterfeit coin in the shape of self-punishment or the

substitution of minor for major virtues, there are those who substitute a minor loyalty. In the devotion of the wife or mother
who sinks her own individuality in that of husband or son and
who finds thus the end and meaning of her life there may be something fine and ennobling. In her, as also in the loyal follower
who devotes himself to some institution or to some finite leader,
we may have also the expression of a higher loyalty. But such
devotion may, and all too often does, become a hindrance to the
full development of all concerned. The devotion to the church
may become the blind and mischievous sectarianism which
thwarts the ends for which the church exists. The loyalty to
country may become the unthinking patriotism which offers its
life on the altar of a cruel and rapacious war-god, or a shortsighted
tyranny which seeks to suppress all liberty of thought and speech.
The mother's devotion may hang as a dead weight around her
son's neck, preventing him from achieving maturity. In other
words, devotion to a finite love object may become a substitute
for that loyalty to the highest which is indispensable to mental
health both personal and social.

Among those who have effected a reorganization of their lives
on a religious basis we find two types of conversion experience.
Most of those we have studied did not involve the impartation
of new teachings or of new loyalties and standards. An individual
already under high tension because of some inner conflict would
happen in at some religious meeting, and through the power of
the music or through some word of the minister the solution
would come. Such a resolution of an inner conflict is clearly on
the basis of loyalties and standards already accepted. It is to be
noted that the cases reported in Begbie's *Twice-born Men* are
almost exclusively of this type. The other type is that in which
some new doctrine is accepted. Among our cases such acceptance
generally follows a period of inner restlessness and groping after
something new and different. A badly adjusted Jew thus becomes
first a Catholic, then an astrologer, and then a spiritist. A Con-
gregationalist who has been very dependent upon her mother,
when the mother dies, takes up with a Pentecostal group and be-

lieves that the Lord is directing her every step. To such cases may be added those obtained especially on the mission fields in the form of proselytes from other religions. We may venture the guess that in addition to the restless group who are seeking insistently for something new there will be those who are won over through the personal influence of the missionary. Personal attachment to the missionary carries with it the acceptance of the missionary's standards.

It is furthermore to be noted that among those who have passed through mystical experiences there are those who emerge with new insights and those in whom the net result is an emotional reinforcement of traditional beliefs. Most of those whom Starbuck studied seem to have been of this latter type; so also the great Roman Catholic mystics. Santa Teresa, after finding convent life rather tedious and stale and profitless, finds it transformed through the experience of illumination and gives herself to a life of untiring and effective activity. But her mystical experiences brought to her no important new insights. Neither did those of Suso or of Madame Guyon. For them the mystical experience merely infused new life and meaning into a dead tradition by connecting it with a vital relationship. There are however those who emerge with new insights and with a more comprehensive understanding. Among these we would certainly place Paul of Tarsus and George Fox and Luther and Ezekiel. We may be fairly sure that Jesus was of this group.

In thus singling out for special consideration in this discussion of sin and salvation the eruptive or cataclysmic type of religious experience, I do not for one instant intend to ascribe to it any peculiar value. The important question is always the result attained in terms of the richness or fullness of life which is to be found through living in harmony with that which is enduring and universal in human experience. It is to be recognized that the cataclysmic type of experience is due usually to the sudden unblocking of that which has been preventing normal development. Its chief value from the standpoint of this inquiry is the light it throws upon the laws and forces involved in spiritual life and development and the significance of the various types of mental illness.

It should furthermore be recognized that the problem of sin and salvation is to a large extent identical with that of mental illness and its cure. The qualification is necessary because it is possible to be very sinful without being mentally ill, as is the case with many delinquents and criminals. It is also possible to be mentally ill without being sinful, as in the case of certain organic diseases and in some who pass through acute upheavals and mutation periods. For the most part, however, what we know as mental illness represents either the crucial or the terminal stage of inner conflicts which arise within those who are trying to serve two masters, those who recognize and accept an ultimate loyalty but have not been able to give up desires and tendencies which belong to an earlier stage of development.

In using the word "sin" I am not unmindful of the disfavor into which it has fallen. Neither do I object to the substitution of new words for old; that I regard as inevitable in the growth of language and culture. I retain the word "sin" because none of the proposed substitutes carries quite the same idea. None of them expresses so exactly what according to our findings is the real evil. It must not be forgotten that the word "sin" implies the rupture of one's supreme loyalties as represented in the idea of God. Our inquiry has led us to the conclusion that right relationship with that which is represented by the idea of God is essential to mental or spiritual health. For the idea of God is the symbol of what is best in the collective interests. It originates, according to the Freudians, in the relationship to the parents and early guides upon whom the young child is dependent for support and affection and it represents to the individual that which is abiding and supreme in his social relationships. By our loyalties to parents and early guides our ethical standards and attitudes are determined, and from them there is no escape except through growth into a higher loyalty and a more comprehensive understanding. The delinquent or the criminal who rebels against these primary loyalties may escape the sense of condemnation within but he is likely to clash with the policeman without. Eventually he will probably meet the policeman within.

Only on the basis of a loyalty to the group and an observance of that which its welfare requires can any society survive. Such observance must be maintained by force if necessary. The task of education is to internalize those laws of life which racial experience has found to be essential to individual and social well-being, and attempts to escape from the inherited loyalties and their associated standards are the source of most of our personal and social evils. We have been led furthermore to the conclusion that only in so far as it is accompanied by the sense of isolation and estrangement does the sense of personal failure and shortcoming lead to mental illness. The recognition of our shortcomings is a precondition of growth and achievement while the basis of all psychotherapy is the removal of the sense of isolation. By restoring the individual to right relationship through confession and forgiveness he is set free to strive for the attainment of his moral objectives. The word " sin " by its implied reference to that which is supreme in one's hierarchy of loyalties thus points to the root of the difficulty, and for the religious worker to follow the psychiatrist in using such substitutes as " maladjustment," " immaturity " or " mental disease " is merely to supply evidence of the increasing tendency toward the secularization of religious work.

On the basis of our findings the essential features in any plan of salvation may be summed up as follows:

1. Commitment to that which is supreme in the hierarchy of loyalties. This involves first acceptance and then transcendence of the primary loyalties. The individual must find his way through the teachings of tradition to some first-hand vision of his own. He must attain to a more comprehensive understanding and to the autonomy that goes therewith. This proposition would seem to hold true no matter what the accepted philosophy of life. For the nonreligious man it would mean the psychoanalytic doctrine of autonomy and maturity. No man is well and no man is grown up until he has emerged from the stage of dependence and has worked out his own philosophy of life so as to be able to stand

on his own feet regardless of outward changes. For the religious man it means the recognition that earthly parents and guides are but representatives of an undying Love to whom he owes allegiance and in whom he must find the meaning of his life.

In the matter of the acceptance of the primary loyalties some reservation should be made with reference to the problem of the adolescent who is in process of finding himself. He often goes through a period of rebellion against the primary loyalties and the tradition in which he has been brought up. It may be maintained, however, that the outcome in his case is going to depend upon the extent to which he is genuinely trying to transcend the early training or to what extent he is merely in search of easy satisfactions and of the rationalizations which will permit them.

2. Thoroughgoing honesty in the facing of the facts. There must be an abandonment of all subterfuges and disguises and the consequent finding of justification and satisfaction in the sense of inner peace and fellowship. This involves the shift in the basis of self-respect from the static to the dynamic morality. It implies the recognition of the principle that ethical codes and values are but functions of the loyalties and that the basis of friendship is to be found not in outward correctness of behavior but in the kinship of loyalty and purpose and in the sharing of experience on the deeper levels. This, as we have seen, was the essence of Paul's discovery regarding the spirit as against the law. It was also the basis of the doctrine of justification by faith which was central in Luther's teaching. It is also the basis of all psychoanalytic therapy.

3. Progressive unification on the basis of accepted loyalties and standards. From the psychotherapeutic standpoint this means that while the physician listens patiently and sympathetically to the patient's difficulties, it is only in order that he may be able to help him toward that transformation of personality which he calls maturity. From the religious point of view it is the old doctrine of sanctification. No matter how imperfect a man may be, he is saved as soon as he is restored to right relationship with God and has joined the ranks of those who are striving to become better. He is thus set free from the sense of estrangement and condemna-

tion, but only that he may strive for the attainment of his true objectives. The perfect Love represented by the idea of God requires of him nothing short of his best. The end of all religion is not states of feeling but the transformation of the personality.

THE NATURE AND FUNCTION OF RELIGION

Our findings give no support to the current view that religion is an "escape from reality." On the contrary, we have found convincing evidence that religious concern is associated with awareness of danger and with attempts to face personal difficulties. It is not characteristic of the concealment and drifting reactions. Even in these cases in which religion enters into a delusional reconstruction we have discovered that it has a constructive function. Not only does it serve to maintain the integrity of the personality but also to preserve a pleasanter and more friendly attitude than the individuals under observation would have been likely to have without it.

Our conclusion is that religion has to do with the organization of personal and social experience. Some sort of philosophy of life, some sort of organization and structuralization of experience we have found to be necessary for every individual if he is to be able to reason and function. This philosophy of life is to be termed religion in so far as it reaches the level of what for the individual concerned are the supreme and enduring loyalties and values. According to Moore, no race has ever been found that did not have some sort of religion. This observation [15] points to the conclusion that no race can survive unless it finds effective means of transmitting and internalizing in the form of conscience those loyalties and values which experience has proved to be important. The test of the worth of any religion or of any ethical system would thus be the extent to which it enabled its adherents to survive in the struggle for existence, and to attain to the abundant life.

It follows therefore that religion is to be regarded as an attempt

---

[15] George Foote Moore, *Birth and Growth of Religion* (New York, Charles Scribner's Sons, 1924), p. 1.

to face and grapple with the realities of life, not to escape from them. It is an attempt to bring personal and group interests into harmony with the universal and to find that upon which one can depend amid the changes and perils of life. But while religion itself is no escape from reality it is nevertheless true that there are multitudes of religious people who are not ready to pay the price of complete commitment and thoroughgoing honesty which true religion demands. Such people do resort to counterfeit coinage and subterfuges of all sorts.

Organized Religion

In our study of acute disturbances we found as one of the characteristic constellation of ideas the conviction of being commissioned to carry out some important task of religious significance. Of our 173 hospital cases 24 thus felt that they had a prophetic message to deliver. In our cases of religious genius they not only had such an idea but they also carried it out. In this fact we have seen evidence of the social roots of religion and of the social requirements of human nature. Just as the delinquent, in order to escape the sense of inner discomfort, must have his gang and seek social validation for his antisocial tendencies, so the man who finds some new insight which seems to him of vital importance feels impelled to share it with his fellows and to give himself to the establishment of the kind of values he has found. It seems to be of the very essence of religion that it must express itself socially. The explanation is that religion has to do with the ongoing process of race perpetuation and improvement and that it looks toward the establishment and making effective of loyalties that are universal. To become truly religious is to commit oneself to that task.

In the Christian church we see those who are bound together by the acceptance of a common loyalty and a common ideal as represented in the life and teachings of Jesus of Nazareth. That loyalty has been transmitted across the ages among men of different races. It has furnished the ideal or standard toward which multitudes have striven. It has been internalized in the form of conscience in countless millions of men and has thus served to develop the common "super-ego" which, according to Freud, is the determinant of a particular culture. Badly split up as it has been through divergent interpretations and the intervention of special loyalties, tragically as it has failed to be true to its founder's teachings, the common allegiance has yet given the stamp to our present civilization.

It should be clearly recognized that the church is a group of persons united by a common loyalty and that the body of doctrines is of secondary importance. The doctrines or standards are commonly accepted because of the loyalties. Most people belong to one church rather than to another because they happen to be born in it. Hence the absurd situation which we find in so many of our American villages with half a dozen small Protestant evangelical churches, each with about the same form of worship, about the same type of otherworldly message, and the same type of gospel songbook. They persist merely because of the family ties which hold over from one generation to another. Herein lies the great weakness of an established religious institution. In the beginning it is composed of those who have had a common vision and have accepted for themselves a common purpose and a common allegiance. But as new generations come on the scene the vision fades and the common tendency is constantly to try to maintain the loyalties at the least possible cost. Those born into the church are all too often unwilling to give that complete devotion which is necessary for growth into full maturity and for attainment of any clear vision of the higher loyalty and its implications. With the passing of the years the church thus becomes cluttered up with all sorts of protective devices, and churches which in the beginning had original and distinctive features tend constantly toward a standardized pattern. Nevertheless the church does provide a seedbed for the prophetic vision and from its ranks come new prophets and leaders.

From the therapeutic standpoint the church at its best is a group of imperfect persons united on the basis of an ideal which they are seeking to realize in their own lives and in the social order. Of all institutions the church, despite its weaknesses and shortcomings, is the one in which men meet on their highest levels, where they confess their weaknesses and sins with the assurance of social understanding and support and yet without any lowering of standards.

PART III

PRACTICAL APPLICATIONS

VIII

WHERE PRIEST AND PHYSICIAN MEET

ACCORDING TO THE Fourth Gospel a blind man once sat by the wayside, begging. They had no institutions in those days and for such unfortunates there was no other means of subsistence. Of those who passed by, the more kindly disposed might toss him a coin. If any stopped to think of the problem he presented they would generally assume in accordance with the prevailing theology that he was atoning for transgressions, either his own or of his parents. We may be sure that anyone in his position would many times ask himself the meaning of it all. Why was he so afflicted? Whose fault was it? Why was he in the world, anyway? We can hardly blame him if he should find the current answers unsatisfactory. Then Jesus passed by, and his disciples, making the usual assumption, inquired: " Rabbi, who did sin, this man or his parents, that he should be born blind? " The answer of Jesus is characteristic. He rejected their assumption and brushed aside the speculation with the reply: "Neither did this man sin nor his parents, but that the works of God should be made manifest in him." He forthwith proceeded to heal him.

In this answer of Jesus we see a fine example of the religious attitude. To him the sight of the blind beggar called for understanding and for action. He was for him a problem to be solved and he saw in him a man who was not without his own reason for existence. Even this unfortunate had a blessing to bestow and a blessing to win.

Certainly the passing centuries have brought a real measure of justification to this ancient saying. Through our efforts to help the sick has come the science of physiology and of medicine. Through our efforts to help the blind has come considerable insight into the laws of learning. Out of the efforts to teach the deaf to speak has come the invention of the telephone which has done so much to annihilate distance and to bring the world together. We are beginning to learn that the society which does not exterminate the unfortunate or leave them to beg by the wayside, finds in its efforts to help them a blessing which returns to itself, not merely in the finer and kindlier spirit which is engendered, but in the discoveries which are made and the laws which are revealed.

In this inquiry we have been exploring the experiences of those who in the time of Jesus were not even allowed to sit by the wayside and beg, but were generally driven out into the desert beyond the city gates. It is my hope that we may in some measure have succeeded in establishing the fact that in them also the works of God are being made manifest, that they too have a message to give to those who have eyes to see and ears to hear, a message concerning the end and meaning of life and the spiritual forces which are involved. I trust that I may now be justified in proceeding on the assumption that in this problem of the mentally ill the provinces of priest and physician meet and that only as the two professional groups join hands, only as we approach this problem from all angles and explore the inner world throughout its entire range will it be possible to give these sufferers any real help or arrive at any true understanding of the meaning of their experiences.

To the medical group it is not necessary for me to offer suggestions. In my capacity as a representative of the patients I may have somewhat to say, but not as a representative of the clergy. The medical men have been on the job and they have made real progress. The care of the mentally ill is still far from what we would like to see, but when we look back and see how far we have come there is cause for real satisfaction.

In the pages that follow I shall address myself chiefly to religious workers. I think I have now shown that, whatever the physical factors which may or may not be involved, the problem of mental illness has to do with the philosophy of life and usually with the sense of personal failure. I think that I have shown that certain types of mental disorder are very closely related to certain types of religious experience and that a consideration of the one throws light upon the other. I have also sought to show that in the experiences of the mentally ill there are operative those profound and delicate laws of the spiritual life with which theology deals. We are thus afforded an approach to these laws, not just through traditional formulae, but through the firsthand study of living human experience. My task now is to examine the service which the church today is actually performing and the trends which are therein revealed; then to make such suggestions as I may be able for increasing its effectiveness in the ministry of the sick of soul.

In thus addressing myself to the religious workers I am guided not merely by the fact that my professional standing is with them, but more especially by the fact that until recently they have been paying little attention to the problem. It seems truly an astounding situation that a group of sufferers larger than that to be found in all other hospitals put together,[1] a group whose difficulties seem to lie for the most part in the realm of character rather than in that of organic disease, should be so neglected by the church. Notwithstanding the fact that the church has always been interested in the care of the sick and that the Protestant churches of America have been supporting 380 or more hospitals,[2] they are giving scarcely any attention to the maladies of the mind. Only three of these 380 hospitals, so far as I am able to discover, concern them-

[1] According to the "Report of the Council on Medical Education and Hospitals" (*Journal of the American Medical Association*, March 7, 1936), the total average population in our American hospitals on December 31, 1935, was 876,689. Of this number 508,448 were in hospitals for nervous and mental disease. It is of course to be remembered that the turnover in these latter institutions is low — only 173,000 admissions in 1935 as compared with 6,868,000 for the general hospitals. It is also to be remembered that these figures include also the mentally deficient.

[2] *World Survey* (New York, Interchurch Press, 1920), I, 246. According to the 1935 "Report of the Council on Medical Education and Hospitals," the total number of church hospitals, including Roman Catholic, is 970. These had 113,268 beds, an average census of 69,592 and an admission rate of 1,950,308.

selves particularly with that problem. The more than 400,000 mental sufferers are being cared for almost entirely in state institutions. Here they are left practically without Protestant religious ministration.[3] The situation which I found in the hospital in which I was a patient is representative. Most state hospitals do have religious services on Sunday. This custom they have accepted in accordance with hoary tradition, and they may even pay the minister a small honorarium. Many superintendents look upon this as good publicity. It helps them to establish local contacts and serves to conciliate and educate influential people. Such services are in my judgment little more than a gesture. Full-time, trained men serving in the capacity of chaplains, other than those now working under the Council for the Clinical Training of Theological Students (see p. 251), are scarcely to be found. Full-time chaplains in prisons and reformatories we do find, but for the mentally ill the practice is to call in ministers from neighboring churches, who know nothing of the special problems of those whom they are thus asked to serve, and who seldom attempt to inform themselves. It seems therefore not inaccurate to say that if a man has a broken leg he can in almost any part of the country be cared for in a church hospital, at church expense, and under church auspices; but if he has a broken heart he is sent to a state institution, there to be forgotten by the church.

I am guided also by my belief in the significance of the problem which is presented in the mentally ill. A distinguished psychologist is accustomed to say that in this problem we have the very storm center of the sciences of psychology, philosophy, religion, medicine and sociology. With this view I am in full agreement. The more I deal with the experiences of the mentally ill, the more I am convinced that in so far as we attain to any true understanding of them, so far shall we be able to see the meaning and end of

[3] In those institutions with which I have been familiar the Roman Catholic church has been more active than the Protestant. They have had some priest especially assigned to the institution. Their activity centers around the administering of the sacraments. They are particularly faithful in performing the last rites to those who are on the " danger list."

human life, both individual and collective. And in so far as we attain to such understanding, we should be well on our way toward building the city of brotherhood and co-operation on the place where the jungle now stands and greed and ruthless competition rule.

IX

THE CHURCH IN ACTION

A Small-Town Parish

For our first task we shall undertake a study of the service which the church is actually performing and of the current trends among the more forward-looking churches. We shall begin with the examination of a small-town parish.

The parish chosen for this study centers in a county seat of about three thousand inhabitants in a good farming section of the Middle West. Agriculture is the chief industry and the village itself is made up of tradesmen, artisans, professional men and laborers who serve the farming population. The early settlers came chiefly from New York and New England. Their descendants still make up the bulk of the population. Those of foreign birth who settled here came chiefly from western and northern Europe. The community has been fairly prosperous although in recent years it has suffered severely from the depression, which has hit the farmers probably harder than any other group. The level of education is high. Most of the present generation of young people are at least highschool graduates and about one in fifteen has college or normal school training.

The Protestant churches in this community are strong. Approximately two-thirds of the adults are church members. This membership is distributed among half a dozen Protestant churches and one small Roman Catholic church. The general region in which the community is located may be regarded as the area of Protestant Christianity's maximum effectiveness.

The church under consideration belongs to the moderately liberal wing of the Protestant group. It has at least for seven years given loyal support to a forward-looking young minister, whose readiness to co-operate, whose balanced judgment, and whose intimate knowledge of his people were the chief reasons for selecting this parish for study.

We may notice first of all that in this much organized community the churches are the institutions in which men meet on their highest levels. There are in the community a number of lodges, composed largely of church people, which in their meetings employ a certain amount of religious ritual and are actuated by motives akin to the religious. They are however secret organizations with a restricted membership and their benevolence is generally limited to their own group. There are also in this community some workers' groups — a farmers' organization and a labor union or two. These also exist for the interests of their particular group. There are likewise several patriotic organizations — an American Legion Post and a D.A.R. The schools of the community, supported by public taxes and controlled by public officers, have as their definite task to induct the young into the experience of the race. In this respect the functions of school and church are similar. It is to be noted that the school was originally a branch of the church and that in many countries church and school are both supported by the state. Under the American plan of separation between church and state it is left to the school to give instruction in the various branches of secular knowledge while the church as a voluntary organization deals with the motivating forces.

In contrast to most other voluntary organizations the church is not restricted in membership nor are its meetings closed or secret. Anyone may attend its meetings, even though he comes to criticize. It is, moreover, built upon the family as a unit. At this church's Sunday morning services about two hundred persons of both sexes and of all ages and social strata, assemble together to consider problems relating to their ultimate destiny both as individuals and in the aggregate, and to bring themselves into an emotional relationship with the God whom they regard as the source of their life, the controller of their destiny, and the one to whom they owe unreserved allegiance. In its activities this church seeks not merely the improvement of the personal and family and community life. It is also concerned with the welfare of the entire world and every year it contributes a not inconsiderable amount of money to the missionary enterprise.

At its best this church service calls forth a deep emotional response. To those who are assembled it brings back tender memories of their loved ones at their best and of those to whom they have most looked up, and it directs their attention back across the centuries to a beautiful and majestic figure. In the historical life and teaching of the church's founder they see the finest expression of the human spirit and the ideal or norm by which they seek to direct their lives. They see this figure of Jesus glorified through his sacrificial death and exalted through the devotion of countless men and women who down through the ages have responded to his call and have given up all that they had for his sake and for that of his cause. All these memories and associations aided by religious symbolism and music can be used with telling effect by the able leader to stir the emotions and wills of his people. Even those who may be half-hearted in their devotion commonly turn to the church in the great crises of life when they find themselves standing on the threshold of the limitless and mysterious unknown. They turn to the church at time of marriage, of birth, and of death, to seek its blessing and support.

The leader of this church is a man of special training. In addition to a broad general education in a college of high standing he has taken the full course in a good professional school. He has made a critical study of the church's sacred book, the Bible; he has surveyed the history of the Christian church; he has informed himself regarding other religions and regarding the philosophy and psychology of religion in general. In the light of these studies he has thought through his own philosophy of life and has taken special interest in the problems relating to personal counseling. This particular pastor, who has now been for seven years in the same field, has won the confidence of his people, not only because of his mastery of the subjects with which he deals in his preaching and teaching, but because of their faith in him as a wise friend and a man of personal integrity and consecration. Many of them come to him with their personal problems. He is in fact in this community the man best equipped to deal with personality difficulties. Of the physicians none has received more than a very brief and formal training in psychiatry, which is apt to be worse than none at all.

With the help of this pastor the attempt was made to classify his people with reference to the type of adjustment they had made. In this study we took the family as the unit and listed all those over twelve years of age regardless of whether their names were on the church rolls. In each case we asked the questions, What is this person's attitude toward the faith of his fathers? Has he sincerely accepted it or has he rejected it? In the latter case, has this rejection been in obedience to a higher loyalty? Or is it merely rebellion and self-assertion and socialization on a lower level? We also asked, What degree of integration has been attained? Is there growth in the direction of inner unification, or is there the attempt to serve two masters? If the latter seems to be the case, are there signs of inner conflict and distress? Is there any resort to the many concealment devices? Our findings were as follows:

1. Classed as growing in the direction of socialization and unification — 186. The pastor felt that these had sincerely accepted for themselves the loyalties and standards represented by the church and were growing in the direction of their accepted ideals. About 80 of this group were young people between the ages of 12 and 20. While they were still immature, he felt that their progress to date had been satisfactory. In this group he placed also several persons who, although not professing Christians or church attendants, were public-spirited and honorable citizens, who were seemingly true to what to them was their highest loyalty.

2. Classed as having a level of adjustment that is merely con-

temporary and local — 207. The pastor felt that their attitude was passive and indifferent. They seemed engrossed in the cares and pleasures of life. They were fairly well adjusted as regards vocation, sex and social life, but they were giving no serious thought to the higher obligations which they had accepted. They were thus serving two masters. If questioned about their religion they would profess allegiance but would show no clear recognition of some rather obvious inconsistencies. In the matter of church attendance those in this group would come occasionally.

3. Classed as " difficult " — 37. This group corresponds to the " isolated " on our chart. It includes those who seemed to their pastor to be maintaining their loyalties and their self-respect by distorting their beliefs and substituting minor for major virtues. Among these he found 11 persons who were constantly complaining and ailing and seeking sympathy, eight who were chronic faultfinders, seven who resorted to excuses and alibis, six who were over-sensitive, four who were religiously fanatical and two who were busybodies and troublemakers.

4. Classed as " distressed " — 21. By " distressed " we meant that they were aware of their inconsistencies to the point of being alarmed over the situation and of seeking a way out. In some of these cases economic and marital difficulties were a factor in upsetting the equanimity. Several were young people who were having difficulty in managing a troublesome sex-drive and bringing it into conformity to their religious ideals.

5. Classed as " pagans " — 30. These were persons who although brought up in church families had disavowed their early loyalties and were comfortable about it. They were mostly " playboys " and " roughnecks " of the near-delinquent sort.

6. Regarded as " down-and-out " — 22. Of these 10 were psychotic, four near-psychotic, and eight delinquent. Of the psychotics four were epileptics, two confirmed alcoholics, two senile cases and two paranoics. Only three of these had been hospitalized. Of the delinquents three are now serving sentences in jails or reformatories.

In making this classification the aim was to look at the situation

from the standpoint of the individual himself as well as from that
of the group in which he had been reared. What the pastor gave
was his estimate of how each person had handled the ideals which
had been implanted through his early training, and his success or
failure in living up to them. This was of course a most delicate
and difficult task, one involving considerable interpretation and
guesswork. In not a few instances however the pastor had been
permitted to see behind the scenes in his efforts to help persons
in distress and he felt that the attempt at classification was of
real help to him because of the questions which it raised and the
need to which it drew his attention.

The outstanding fact revealed through this study was the potency of home influences in the determination of ideals, and the
infrequency of cases in which these influences were transcended.
The importance of home influences is revealed in a study of the
relationship between the adjustments of the children and those
of the parents. We found in this community 182 persons over 12
years of age whose parents also had been observed and classified.
Of these, 69 were in class 1. The fathers were distributed as follows: class 1, 20 per cent; class 2, 49 per cent; class 3, 14 per cent;
the rest unknown. The mothers were distributed: class 1, 54 per
cent; class 2, 25 per cent; class 3, 10 per cent; and the rest unknown.

Of the 182 persons 33 were maladjusted. That is, they belonged
in classes 3, 4, 5 and 6. Of these maladjusted individuals the
fathers were rated as follows: class 1, 3 per cent; class 2, 24 per
cent; class 3, 10 per cent; class 4, 14 per cent; class 5, 33 per cent;
the rest unknown. Of the mothers the ratings were: class 1, 6 per
cent; class 2, 33 per cent; class 3, 37 per cent; the rest unknown.

We thus note that in the case of the children rated in class 1
only 14 per cent of the fathers and 10 per cent of the mothers
were rated as maladjusted and none of these were in class 5. In
the case of the maladjusted children 58 per cent of the fathers and
37 per cent of the mothers were rated as maladjusted.

Approaching the problem from the standpoint of the parents'
adjustments we find in our group of 182, 50 mothers and 19

fathers who had been rated in class 1. There were eleven cases in which both parents were rated in class 1. Of these cases the children were also rated in class 1 in 75 per cent of the cases in which the mothers were in class 1 and in 73 per cent of the cases in which the fathers were rated in class 1. Of those cases in which both parents were in class 1 all but one of the children were also in class 1.

In these 182 cases there were 50 maladjusted fathers and 53 maladjusted mothers. In 37 cases both parents were maladjusted. The adjustments of the children in these cases were as follows:

Maladjusted fathers: class 1, 12; class 2, 22; class 3, 3; class 4, 4; class 5, 9.

Maladjusted mothers: class 1, 8; class 2, 28; class 3, 4; class 4, 4; class 5, 9.

Both parents maladjusted: class 1, 4; class 2, 18; class 3, 3; class 4, 4; class 5, 8.

While the data provided by this study are entirely too meager to permit us to speak with any great degree of assurance, they are quite in line with what we might anticipate. They indicate that the children tend very strongly to take over the ideals of their parents. Where the parents have recognized those loyalties and obligations for which the church stands and are growing in the direction of unification on that basis, the children likewise tend to fall into the same group. It is an interesting fact that in those cases in which the parents were maladjusted this tendency, while clear, was far less pronounced. Apparently the church group had not been without a corrective and wholesome influence.

Very striking was the small number of those who were intelligently atheistic or agnostic. There were few who in sincerity and good faith had thought their way through to a divergent view. The reasons advanced for nonattendance or disinterest in the church seemed to be for the most part rationalizations. There were the ever present number who are unable to see beyond the hypocrisy of church members, seeking thus to maintain their own self-respect by belittling others. There were also those who made light of religion and of the church, thus making use of the common devices of jesting and derision. There were also those who had shifted their loyalties. But the great majority seemed to fall into class 2, those who do not consciously break with the faith of their fathers but who become increasingly indifferent and absorbed in other interests.

THE EFFECT OF RELIGIOUS LIBERALIZATION UPON THE INFLUENCE OF THE CHURCH

The small number of the intelligently atheistic or agnostic was a fact that impressed me in a study which I made about twenty years ago of rural church attendance in five different regions of the United States. This study [1] which was made for the most part under the direction of the Presbyterian Board of Country Church Work, dealt with one county in western Tennessee, with northeastern Missouri, northeastern Kansas, Westchester County, New York, and with four communities in western Maine. The basis was a total of about 12,000 persons. The findings showed a marked falling off in church attendance in the liberalized areas as compared with the conservative. Thus in western Tennessee, a very conservative section, I found only about 20 per cent of the heads of families who were classed by their neighbors among the non-churchgoers. In Missouri 28 per cent of all those over fifteen years old were so rated. In Kansas the percentage of non-churchgoers was 42, in New York 53, and in Maine 65. The one factor which seemed to vary directly with this marked decrease in church attendance was the liberalization of popular religious opinion. Not only was the influence of the church least in the more liberalized areas but even here the more conservative groups were holding their people better than the liberal.

It was found that the falling off in church attendance was greatest among the less educated classes. Among these I discovered little frank skepticism. The majority of those who did not go to church gave no clearly defined reasons for not going. They believed that the church was a good thing. They liked to see their

---

[1] " Factors Which Have to Do With the Decline of the Country Church," *American Journal of Sociology*, Sept., 1916.

children go. They had simply become indifferent. With the liberalization of popular religious opinion which is breathed in from the social atmosphere, the old fear compulsions lose their power and the old belief in the efficacy of going to church as a means of salvation is challenged by the assertion, " I'm as good as Smith and he goes to church." In so far as such men even in the more liberalized sections could express their religious views, these views would usually be of older theology. The religious atmosphere had merely made less real the beliefs to which they still adhered and had brought forward no other compelling appeal.

The same study revealed that of the men active in community affairs in seven liberalized communities 73 per cent were church members, and that of those not active in the church nearly 80 per cent were engaged in no organized social activity. Those upon whom the church had lost its hold were for the most part no longer interested in anything except their own families, their own work, or their own pleasures.

We thus see that the influence of the church is associated with the solidarity of the family and with the service of the community and that according to this study the men upon whom the church has lost its hold are for the most part lost to organized social activity. We may say that in the process of liberalizing religious opinion the efficiency of the schools and even of the churches themselves has worked at least temporarily to the church's disadvantage. It is not without significance that the better educated and the more public spirited were still for the most part active in the church.

CURRENT TRENDS IN LIBERAL CHURCH WORK

In the twenty years which have elapsed since this study was made the process of liberalization has gone on fairly rapidly, especially in the cities and educational centers. My impression is that the drift away from the churches has likewise been increasing, but I know of no current studies which would furnish the basis for a comparison. A study which has been in process somewhat intermittently by some of my students during the past three years may serve to indicate what is now taking place among liberal religious groups in and around Chicago. It may suggest an explanation of the liberal church's failure to hold its people.

A tendency toward secularization of religious work appears to be the outstanding feature of the present-day situation. This seems due to the shift from the old faith in a revealed religion to an empirical basis. It is shown in a flight into activities — educational, recreational, social — and a discontinuance or curtailment of pietistic religious expression. This is strikingly exemplified in the work of the Y.M.C.A. Beginning in 1844 as a group of young men banded together on a definitely religious basis with a strong evangelistic emphasis which continued on through the beginning of the present century, the Y.M.C.A. has now, especially in the cities, been forced to abandon most of its religious work. The city of Chicago thus has no religious work secretary either in the men's or the women's organization, the old Sunday afternoon religious service has been discontinued, and religion has to be smuggled in under the name of philosophy or psychology. One large Y.M.C.A. center thus has some three hundred group meetings each month, but these consist entirely of educational, recreational and physical training activities. They have no religious meetings for the simple reason that they can no longer get anyone to come. The same tendency is found also in the liberal churches. Among these the Sunday morning religious service still remains the focal point of all activities, but aside from this and from the church school we find the same general tendency which is found in the Y.M.C.A. The old midweek prayer meeting has in most churches been discontinued and the Sunday evening service, if not likewise discontinued, has suffered a change of character. Where formerly it was evangelistic in its tenor, the minister may now give a book review or a lecture on psychology or current events. Sometimes it is transformed into a public forum or replaced by a musical vesper service. In the meantime the number of organizations and activities is being greatly increased and many churches are doing a vigorous institutional work.

The trend toward secularization is shown also in a changing

vocabulary which avoids many of the old symbols and phrases. Instead of the word " God " there is a tendency to use adjectives and circumlocutions. The old word " sin " is in certain circles especially in disfavor. In its place we hear the word " maladjustment." Neither is it customary today in liberal churches to speak of " saving souls " or of " evangelistic work." Instead we hear much of " personal counseling " or " personnel work " or " case work."

Meanwhile we see an increasing emphasis upon programs of social service, of mental hygiene, of social reform, while the old commanding summons to complete commitment to an ultimate loyalty is no longer sounded and religious conversion experiences of the type described by Starbuck are seldom encountered in liberal churches. Out of nineteen liberal churches with an aggregate membership of perhaps fifteen thousand no clear-cut cases were reported for the past year of sudden transformations of character attended by the sense of illumination and mystical identification. Few troubled consciences are today being brought to the liberal minister. The problems that do come are mainly those of economic distress, child guidance, and marital difficulty. Most ministers do have quite a number of conferences relating to commitment to the Christian life, but they approach this problem generally from the common-sense standpoint and do not often come to close grips with fundamental problems of the individual.

In the meantime a new professional group has come upon the scene, the psychiatrists and the psychoanalysts, who are taking over precisely those problems which have been most distinctively the church's own. The specialists in medical psychology are rapidly becoming the Protestant confessors. In our larger centers, at least, it is they who today are most frequently consulted regarding the inner conflicts of modern man. And they are able to give real help. They have, as we have shown, made a systematic and co-operative attack upon problems involved in the breakdown of the personality, and the approach through the study of the pathological has yielded some important new insights into the laws of the spiritual life. Their point of view is however not that of the minister of religion. Few among them have brought to bear upon these disorders of the personality the insights which come from an understanding of the ultimate loyalties and values with which religion deals.

We were impressed also by the evidence of a decreasing assurance on the part of religious workers regarding their aims and their techniques. Having accepted the findings of modern science and having given up the authority of their own religious tradition, they have no ground of their own to stand on. Their position is often apologetic. They are engaged in explaining ancient tenets in terms of modern thought. Too often they have given up the authority of tradition without having given up the traditional point of view. They are still inclined to begin with the past rather than with the present, with the general rather than with the particular, with books rather than with living human experience, and even in our best theological schools the empirical disciplines are not yet part of the basic structure of theological education. The note of conviction and authority is therefore gone and many liberal clergymen are taking over on authority as part of the gospel of enlightenment the new discoveries of science in the domain of the unconscious without going on to explore this territory for themselves.

THE CHALLENGE TO LIBERAL CHRISTIANITY

The waning influence of liberal Christianity is indeed a cause for serious concern in this period when the world is in transition and needs its message as never before. Modern science has today placed in our hands undreamed-of power and has made our world wonderfully compact. A message can today be sent around the entire globe in less time than one hundred years ago it could be carried across a New England village. Today one can travel around the entire world in less time than it would have taken to journey from the Hudson to the Mississippi one hundred years ago. Machines today do work which then would have required a thousand hands. Such facts are a commonplace. It is only necessary for us in this inquiry to recognize that this mechanical development has not been accompanied by any corresponding social development. We are today as children playing with matches near a powder magazine, or as a boy of five at the wheel of a high-powered motorcar. The very power science has placed in our hands is a source of difficulty and danger. Because our economic system is still based upon the law of the jungle and functions properly only when there is not enough to go around, we are today treated to the absurd spectacle of suffering and even starvation in a land of superabundant plenty. Because we are still ruled by the law of the jungle, nations are still at war with nations and the power of the machine may easily be used to destroy the civilization that has produced it. That love shall reign among men and that truth and righteousness and justice shall prevail has today become no mere visionary utopia. It is rather a stern and imperative necessity if we and our civilization are not to perish from the earth.

The Christian church of today is indeed an army that has suffered serious defeat and part of the lack of confidence responsible for its waning influence is a consequence of the inevitable discouragement and loss of prestige which has resulted from that defeat. Nevertheless there are hopeful elements in the situation. The decreasing assurance of religious workers in regard to their aims and their techniques may represent the giving up of dogmatism and the beginning of that humility which is a precondition of entrance into any kingdom of heaven. Such a period of transition involves inevitable loss. Without the aggressive, enthusiastic conviction on the part of both leaders and people that they have the keys to that which is supremely worth while in life the church cannot be a going concern.

The breaking down of the traditional authority of the church cannot but result in a lessening of its influence and in a disruption of old moral safeguards. But the hands of the clock cannot be turned back. Forces are at work which are beyond our control, the forces of the truth which sets men free. Even though the conservative attitude might succeed in holding the lines a little longer, it offers no solution. The solution lies not in cleaving to the old but in going forward with the advance of truth. In fact, I am inclined to think that the weakness of the liberal group lies precisely in the fact that it has not yet gone far enough. It has merely surrendered the authority of tradition without freeing itself from the traditional point of view. For this reason I hold that the shift from faith in a revealed religion to an empirical basis, which is responsible for so much of the present confusion, must be not merely accepted but eagerly furthered. It is furthermore my conviction that the remaking of the outer world and the cure of the desperate sickness which now threatens to destroy our civilization is inseparably associated with the problems of the inner world and that out of the efforts to understand and help the mentally distressed should come a new vision of the great Reality to whom we give the name of God, in whom alone we are to find the end and meaning of personal and social life and the sources of power and of renewal.

X

FOUNDATIONS OF SPIRITUAL HEALING

In venturing to use the term " spiritual healing " I am probably
laying myself open to criticism. Only a few weeks ago I was
taken severely to task for using the term " cure of souls." A professor of religious education thought it most unfortunate that I
should cling to such an outworn and misleading word as " soul,"
while a psychiatrist friend suggested that it would be much wiser
if I should avoid the use of words like " cure," to which the
medical profession laid an exclusive claim. I am afraid the present title will be open to the same objections.

Now I have no desire to become involved in any controversy
over the use of words and I should be happy to substitute another
phrase if I could find it. I am concerned only to follow out the
logical consequences of our findings as regards the distinctive task
of the clergyman and the conditions essential to its accomplishment. We have found that mental illness of the functional type
has to do with the philosophy of life and usually with the sense
of personal failure. We have arrived at the conclusion that acute
upheavals are really attempts at reorganization which are closely
related to those eruptive solutions of inner conflicts so familiar to
the religious worker under the name of " conversion experiences."
We have furthermore concluded that in mental illness there are
operative those profound and delicate laws of the spiritual life
with which theology deals. If our findings are correct it follows
that the religious worker, as his major problem, is dealing with
precisely those same inner adjustments and conflicts which come

within the province of the psychiatrist. It is of course true that he is dealing with these difficulties in their incipient rather than in their terminal stages. But that only makes his task the more important. If only he have understanding, there is no one who has it in his power to do more effective preventive work than the minister who in his professional capacity goes in and out among his people, visiting them in their homes, talking with them individually about their personal problems, and preaching from his pulpit on that which has to do with the end and meaning of life. For the same reason, if he have not understanding, he may be worse than ineffective. He may do actual harm. But the fact remains that so long as the church is in existence and so long as it retains any influence whatsoever, the minister will be engaged in the same general task as the psychiatrist. Regardless of the name we use, for better or for worse, he will be doing psychotherapeutic work. It would seem advisable that this fact should be recognized and that he should be enabled to do his rightful part toward the achievement of mental health among those whom he serves.

I count it, therefore, as not the least important of my obligations as a student of the advanced disorders of the personality that I should do my part toward acquainting ministers generally with the insights derived from dealing with serious mental illness. In endeavoring to perform this task before groups of ministers I have not infrequently encountered among them a certain impatience. They want to be told at once what to do. They want rules of procedure which they can apply and they are apt to be restive under the attempt to discover the meaning of the different forms of mental illness.

For such an attitude there is much justification.[1] The driver of an automobile does not have to be a physicist or even a mechanic and an electrician may be perfectly competent for a practical task even though he may think of electricity in terms of " juice." One does not need to understand all the factors involved in order to do good psychotherapeutic work. In fact, much research work hav-

---

[1] Cf. Cabot and Dicks, *The Art of Ministering to the Sick* (New York, Macmillan Co., 1936), pp. 49–50.

ing to do with the treatment of the mentally ill has arrived at
erroneous conclusions just because it has not taken this principle
into account. The results obtained with dementia praecox patients by one set of workers through the treatment of " focal in-
fections " (see above, pp. 100–1) or through the inoculation with
horse serum do not prove the validity of their respective theories.
Other workers, using the same methods, arrive at different results.
Apparently the results obtained have been due to other factors,
such as the physician's faith in his own remedy, the greater amount
of attention bestowed upon sufferers who had before been
neglected and the consequent change in spiritual atmosphere.
Neither does the fact that important beneficial results are secured
through psychoanalytic treatment prove the correctness of psychoanalytic theories. The fact is that psychotherapy is far less
dependent upon technique than it is upon the personal relationship between physician and patient. Wherever the patient has
come to trust the physician enough to unburden himself of his
problems and wherever the physician is ready to listen with
intelligent sympathy, good results are likely to follow regardless
of the correctness or incorrectness of the physician's particular
theories or procedures. This principle has been stated by Dr.
Macfie Campbell in an article which ought to be in the hands of
every physician and clergyman. Says Dr. Campbell in part:

> The essence of psychotherapy, no matter what the special procedure may
> be, is that Brown, an individual in trouble, is getting an honest chance to
> bring up important problems of his life before McConnachie, the physician,
> who is willing to listen to him, and that McConnachie is honestly en-
> deavoring to pool his special knowledge with Brown's lay experience to
> see whether poor Brown can by means of his help make a better job of his
> life and get along without his previous evasive reactions, whether the latter
> consist of physical symptoms, special fears, domestic friction, economic in-
> efficiency, or social eccentricities. . . .
> So long as McConnachie is intelligent and listens long enough to the
> information which Brown can put before him, and so long as he is able
> to talk to Brown in a useful and constructive way, details of procedure are
> of vanishing importance. One physician may wish to employ the dramatic
> technique of the hypnotic procedure in order that he may listen to Brown
> and talk to Brown. Brown may be docile and have no objections to this

little drama. In fact the mild mystery connected with it may somewhat exalt McConnachie in his eyes. Or he may find it less embarrassing to tell some things with head averted or with eyes closed. It is gratifying to have at the same time the possibility of unburdening and the official fiction that we ourselves are not really conscious of the facts we are disclosing. So in diplomacy it is sometimes useful to communicate certain information but at the same time to make a " dementi officiel." This is in accord with diplomatic tradition and the diplomatist maintains his self-respect. . . .

An orthodox follower of Freud may prefer to sit behind his patient, who lies stretched out on a couch and with closed eyes talks to the physician about whatever happens to come into his or her mind. Here too the patient has an opportunity to talk with averted face and it may be more pleasant for the physician not to have the patient scrutinizing his face for an hour continuously. This setting too may give both to the patient and to the physician a diluted magical feeling which heightens the prestige of the physician.

The essential fact about the situation is that Brown, whether in the hypnotic or in the psychoanalytic setting or sitting with eyes wide open on any convenient chair, is talking seriously and earnestly about vital issues to McConnachie, who is seated upon some equally indifferent article of furniture, but who is profoundly convinced of the important rôle played in many ailments by the complications of human nature and the difficulties of adjustment to a modern cultural environment.[2]

This does not mean that technique is unimportant. There is certainly much to be learned from the experience of successful practitioners which will help in avoiding difficulties and finding useful devices and methods of procedure. From the experienced and skilled worker the novice may learn much about the importance of keeping accurate records. From him he may learn the elements of a good case record and the distinction which, all too often, is not made between the systematic combing over of the ground and the artistic case summary or the record intended for teaching purposes, in which the significant facts are singled out and thrown into clear relief. From the skilled worker the beginner may learn how important it is in questioning a patient or his relatives to establish a proper point of contact. He may note how such a worker begins by putting the informant at ease, how he asks first questions of central interest and works from them

[2] " Psychotherapy," *Boston Medical and Surgical Journal*, Sept. 17, 1925.

back to the questions regarding grandfather or grandmother or the alcoholic uncle, and how carefully he prepares the way for those questions on which the informant is likely to be sensitive. He may learn to recognize the significance of things that are not said and to take note of the sudden pause, of the embarrassed smile, of the averted eyes, or the shift in position which, to those who have eyes to see, may speak as plainly as words. He may learn also the importance of leaving the patient free to tell his own story in his own way with only such questions and comments as are necessary to stimulate him and draw him out and guide him toward the more significant topics.

Probably there is no more important lesson for the average minister or teacher than this art of listening, for not uncommonly he likes to do the talking himself. From the good psychiatrist he should learn the need of beginning with the other fellow, of listening without condemning, of trying to understand his language, particularly that symbolic language which is intended to be understood only by those who have eyes to see and ears to hear. And seeing back of symptom and symbol to the real needs and the unspoken longings, the man of understanding will be little concerned about creed or formula but will concern himself with the task of leading the sufferer in terms of his own formulations to discover for himself that solution of his problem which is socially acceptable and constructive.

While it is necessary to bear in mind the primary importance of the imponderable and elusive personal factors, we should not fail to recognize that there are different psychotherapeutic techniques, each with its particular point of view and its particular uses.

The methods which in the past have generally been employed by the church belong in the " faith healing " group. This form of psychotherapy is characterized by the fact that it relies chiefly upon suggestion. It takes the patient as he is, making little or no attempt to discover the roots of his difficulty, and directs his attention to comforting and constructive thoughts through prayer, friendly advice and devotional books. It would do the church serious injustice not to recognize that considerable good sense has been brought to bear by individual workers and that rather generally a great deal of stress has been placed on facing the facts and squaring accounts and correcting misunderstandings. But there has never been any systematic attempt at treatment on the basis of diagnosis, while in such forms as Christian Science suggestion is even carried to the point of denying the reality of evil and pain and asserting the absolute omnipotence of Mind and Love and Truth.

A somewhat different form of faith healing is that which some years ago received much publicity through M. Coué and his little formula about " getting better and better." Still another is that which makes use of hypnosis. With the patient in the hypnotic condition the practitioner makes constructive suggestions. Of recent years the use of deep hypnosis has been limited. The tendency among those who use hypnosis at all is merely to give suggestions to the patient while the latter is in relaxed condition or under light hypnosis. It is also used for exploratory purposes in order to discover hidden causes of trouble. The disfavor with which hypnosis is now regarded is due to the view that results secured with its help, while often striking, are not permanent. They are suggestions imposed from without and may even tend to weaken the patient's will.

The results secured at religious revivals in the years gone by have undoubtedly been due largely to the influence of suggestion; so also the cures effected at such shrines as Lourdes and Ste. Anne de Beaupré.

A very interesting method is that of moral re-education as represented by Dr. Dubois at the beginning of the present century. He sought to understand the patient's difficulties and to inculcate a morality based on sound rational and biological principles. In this country the moral re-education plan is best represented in the work of Dr. Riggs at Stockbridge, Massachusetts.

The form of psychotherapy now most in the public eye is psychoanalysis. This in its aims is the exact opposite of faith healing. It has often been compared by its proponents to surgery, and major surgery at that. It is an attempt to lay bare and bring into clear consciousness the disowned sexual desires and cravings which it assumes have become detached from the conscious self and are responsible for the neurotic symptoms. Its aim is to make over the harsh conscience and the rigid ethical standards which have led to the disowning of these sex cravings so as to permit of their incorporation in the personality. To this end the psychoanalyst tries to get his patient to live through again his early experiences. The entire procedure is designed to detach the patient from his early loyalties in order to enable him to build up a new philosophy of life in which the dissociated cravings may be properly assimilated. The analysis begins with the understanding that the patient is to tell everything without evasion or concealment. He is required to report his dreams. He is asked for his earliest memories. He is placed in a reclining position and told to report everything that comes into his mind, no matter what it is. All this is done with the assurance that there is to be no moral condemnation. The patient is in fact encouraged to lay bare even the crudest and most primitive sex imaginings. The analyst's task is to listen in a detached and impersonal fashion and to help the patient work out his own solution. It is insisted that the analyst himself must make no suggestions. Particularly must he avoid any imposing of his own standards.

Great stress was in the beginning laid upon the idea of " catharsis." Confession served to let the poisons out of the system and therein lay the curative value of the analysis. It is now recognized that it is not the mere confession which effects the cure but the socialization. The cure is only effected in so far as the sufferer tells his real difficulties to someone whom he trusts, someone who stands to him as the prototype of the father and the representative of authority and who yet is able to hear the worst without condemning him. The importance of this relationship between physician and patient Freud has recognized from the beginning in his doctrine of the "transference." According to this doctrine, in all cases in which the physician is able to accomplish anything it is to be expected that an emotional attachment will develop.[8] This attachment may even go so far as to become a love

---

[8] See above, p. 161, note 8.

relationship. Even so, it is to be accepted and utilized as part of the process of treatment. It must however be broken up before the cure is completed. This is done by analyzing the relationship itself. This task is however a delicate and difficult one and many an analysis has gone on the rocks at just this point.

Jung has taken sharp issue with Freud in this as well as in several other particulars. According to him the physician should seek from the beginning to avoid such complications by directing the patient's attention to that which is beyond himself.[4] He is also inclined to challenge the wisdom of seeking to detach the patient from his early loyalties and attempting to make over his scale of values. Instead of trying to destroy the " super-ego," in order to bring about a synthesis with the disowned elements, Jung is intent upon discovering what the " collective unconscious " wants. He then tries to effect a synthesis between this and the conscious self.[5]

This brief résumé of the chief psychotherapeutic techniques will suffice to indicate that common to them all is the primary importance of the relationship between physician and patient. The techniques and methods of procedure are, as Dr. Campbell points out, of vanishing importance compared with the qualities of heart and mind, the genuine interest in the patient and his problems, together with the balanced judgment and insight and tact necessary to win the patient's confidence and establish the rapport which is the *sine qua non* of all effective psychotherapeutic work. With these qualities the techniques will take care of themselves. Without them good technique may perhaps keep the patient from being disillusioned. This résumé will also serve to indicate that among the various techniques there are two contrasting methods. One of these relies upon personal influence alone in that it seeks to impose suggestions. The other calls also for the discovery and the solving

[4] For an illuminating discussion of this point see Cabot and Dicks, *The Art of Ministering to the Sick,* chap. 12; also, Elwood Worcester, *Body, Mind, and Spirit* (Boston, Marshall Jones, 1931), Introduction.

[5] For Jung's position read his *Modern Man in Search of a Soul* (New York, Harcourt, Brace & Co., 1934), chaps. 2, 3, 6, 11; also his *Two Essays in Analytical Psychology* (New York, Dodd, Mead & Co., 1928).

of the patient's actual difficulties. It seems hardly necessary to say that the hope of genuine progress lies with the latter group.

In the matter of training for psychotherapeutic work it is obvious that in the case of those techniques which rely merely upon personal influence and suggestion there can be no particular type of training which is to be regarded as essential, and that men without any training at all may be quite effective provided only they have the personal qualifications necessary to win confidence and prestige. It is equally clear that for those techniques which call for understanding the training can hardly be too thorough.

In this country the field of psychotherapy is claimed exclusively by the medical profession and no man is considered equipped to deal even with less serious mental disorders unless he has passed through the educational machine leading to the medical degree. Among the psychoanalysts, who have probably done most toward laying the foundations for a true understanding of these disorders, there is a difference of opinion on this matter. Professor Freud himself has come out definitely in favor of "lay analysis."[6] This is not because he wants to lower the standards but because he recognizes the inadequacy of the conventional medical training in the field of mental illness. Adler and Rank seem chiefly interested in the application of the insights derived from psychoanalysis to the field of education, while Jung is frank to say that most of the problems brought to him have to do with the philosophy of life and with religion and that the clergyman ought to be equipped to deal with them, as today he is not.

There can be no question but that membership in the medical profession is today of very great advantage to anyone who wishes to practice psychotherapy. It unlocks the doors. It carries with it a certain prestige; most people today are probably more disposed to unburden themselves to a physician than they are to a clergyman. More than that, there are of course many cases in which organic disease is actually a primary factor and always there is the interaction between the physical and the mental. But once the or-

6 *The Problem of Lay Analysis* (New York, Brentano's, 1927).

ganic factors have been ruled out it seems beside the point whether a man be called a physician or a clergyman or by other title when it comes to intelligent dealing with the emotional and spiritual difficulties of his fellows.   The first essential is that the beams should have been removed from his own eyes.   He should first of all have found solutions for his own difficulties which are socially acceptable in order that his own biases and protective devices may not make him a blind leader of the blind.   He must, in other words, have attained to some measure of discipline and integrity and fineness of character.   Of equal importance is it that he should have checked his own experience and insights in the light of the experiences and insights of others than himself, particularly of the noblest and best in the experience of the race.   A further important requirement is firsthand acquaintance with the primary sources of all knowledge of human nature, the living documents themselves, particularly the revealing documents which are opened in the inner day of judgment.

In these particulars we find a striking contrast between the training of the medical man and that of the clergyman.   The medical man is trained to deal at first hand with living human nature. He knows particularly the dangers and diseases to which flesh is heir, and if he be a psychiatrist, he knows the vagaries of the human spirit.   He has not, however, as an essential part of his training, been introduced to human nature at its best.   In the case of the clergyman the primary stress is laid upon character and purpose and he is introduced in his training to the noblest experiences of the race and to its most important insights.   As yet however it is not an essential part of his training that he should be introduced under guidance to the raw material of life or that he should learn to recognize and understand experiences that are morbid or pathological.

Now I have no brief for either profession.   I have had almost as much difficulty with the one as with the other.   I can only say that from the standpoint of the mentally ill, in whose behalf I speak, I scarcely know which is worse, to have to depend upon a clergyman who has never come to close grips with the realities of human nature, or to be at the mercy of a physician who has no understanding of the spiritual needs and aspirations and of the nobler potentialities of mankind. I am merely convinced that our present system of training experts in the maladies of the personality is in need of improvement. I regard it as a great misfortune that the rigid standardization which now prevails in medical education makes it impossible for a man to qualify as a psychiatrist except by taking five years of expensive and arduous training in order to qualify as internist and surgeon and obstetrician before he can even touch the field of his real interest.[7] I am equally certain that certain things all-important to any true understanding of mental illness have been left out of that conventional training and that constant emphasis upon the organic and the sexual may even distort the vision, when it comes to dealing with the delicate inner adjustments of men, particularly with their philosophy of life and with their religious problems and aspirations.

As for the clergyman, in so far as he has no message for the soul that is sick and no understanding of those experiences in which men are grappling with the issues of spiritual life and death, I am very sure that he will hardly be able to speak with authority regarding the way either to individual or to social salvation. Medical education does stand for one essential requirement. That requirement is firsthand experience under guidance with people that are sick. In the case of the maladies of the personality this would mean that no man is fitted to deal with the incipient disorders of the mind without a background of experience with mental illness of the full-blown variety.

For those who seek authority I am afraid this chapter may not be satisfying. Not in any revelation handed down from the past, not in anything that can be demonstrated in test-tube or under the microscope, not in systems found in books, nor in rules and techniques taken over from successful workers would I seek the basis of spiritual healing, but in the living human documents in all their complexity and in all their elusiveness and in the tested insights

---

[7] Cf. William Healy, " The Newer Psychiatry: Its Field — Training for It." *American Journal of Psychiatry*, Jan., 1926.

of the wise and noble of the past as well as of the present. To the ability to read these human documents in the light of the best human understanding there is no royal road. It calls for that which is beyond anything that books or lectures or schools can impart and to which only a few can attain.

XI

CLINICAL EXPERIENCE IN THE SERVICE
OF THE MENTALLY ILL

ALMOST FROM THE beginning of the specialized religious ministration to the mentally ill, upon which I have been engaged during
the last twelve years, I have been concerned in a plan for the clinical training of theological students. In introducing this plan I
was guided first of all by the conviction which came to me through
my experience as a patient regarding the significance of the experiences of the mentally ill for the student of religion. I was
guided furthermore by the view that the theological schools offered
the strategic point of attack in any attempt to enlist the church
in the service of this group of sufferers and in any attack upon the
problems which they represent. I had, moreover, watched with
interest the medical internes who came to the hospital to work
under guidance as part of their medical training. I had seen how
real, how vital, such instruction became as they and their teachers
dealt together with the actual raw material of life, and I had become convinced that the theological student might well spend less
time with his books and more with the human documents found
in a mental hospital. I had become convinced that clinical experience should be just as important to the man who is to be charged
with the cure of souls as it is to the man who is to care for the
bodies of men.

   This plan for providing clinical training to students of theology,
which began in 1925 with four students at the Worcester State
Hospital, has grown and the movement has been incorporated

under the name of the Council for the Clinical Training of Theological Students. During the present summer some sixty theological students are receiving training at nine different training centers under the auspices of the Council.

Among those who have so generously supported this undertaking there have been divergent and sometimes conflicting points of view on matters that are by no means unimportant. There have been those who flatly reject the psychogenic interpretation of mental illness, represented in this book, and who would explain it rather in terms of organic disease.[1] But in one thing all have agreed. We must begin not with traditions and not with systems formulated in books, but with the open-minded exploration of living human experience in order from that to build up a body of generalizations.

While this project began with the service of the mentally ill, and while the great majority of our students go first to a mental hospital, the scope of the undertaking has been broadened to include other of the infirmities of mankind, such as are concentrated in our prisons, reform schools, child guidance clinics, general hospitals and almshouses. It is our plan to provide adequate supervision of these students not just by placing them in the care of the present type of specialist; we insist upon the guidance of someone who is engaged in exploring these fields of human experience from the specific angle of the student of religion. We are concerned to get light upon the causation, upon the treatment, and upon the implications of such experiences for the problems and laws with which theology is concerned. Without such supervision it is our policy not to open any new center.

Although the scope of our undertaking has thus been broadened to include other forms of human misery, I myself remain an unreconstructed believer in the primacy of the claims of the mentally ill upon the student of religion. This claim rests, as I see it, upon the number of sufferers involved, upon the strange indifference which the church has hitherto shown toward them, and upon the

---

[1] E.g., Dr. Richard C. Cabot, who did much toward launching the project. See his *Art of Ministering to the Sick,* pp. 6–7, 154–6.

peculiar significance of the problems they present. In saying this I do not fail to recognize the importance of other fields. No one can read the account of the work which Mr. Dicks is doing at the Massachusetts General Hospital without feeling the challenge which it brings. He is doing a masterly job of applying the resources of the Christian religion to the needs of the physically ill, and Dr. Cabot in their book [2] has made an important contribution to the religious interpretation of this realm of experience. It is to be noted that Mr. Dicks is concerned chiefly with the problem of technique. The Christian faith he takes for granted, as in his particular task it is right and proper that he should. In the case of the mental sufferer, on the other hand, nothing can be taken for granted. His inner world has gone to pieces or it has been twisted out of shape. The culture patterns in which he was brought up no longer hold good and he questions everything. In so far, therefore, as we are to begin with his experiences and learn to see through his eyes, we must re-examine the foundations of all religious faith and learn to understand the laws and the forces which are involved in his experience. Herein lies the challenge of this problem to the student of religion, especially in this era of transition and change in religious attitudes and beliefs. It calls upon him for something more than alleviation and comfort. It challenges him to discover in the experiences of his patients the operations of that same power that makes for health which Dr. Cabot has found in the human body and described so beautifully. In the measure that we are able to do this, we should have not merely the means of helping many mental sufferers but also a message for all mankind regarding the end and meaning of life.

Our purpose is however not just that of exploration. We are seeking always to relieve human distress and to train the young minister in the fine art of helping those who are in trouble. We hold that service and understanding go ever hand in hand. Without true understanding there can be no effective service in that which concerns the spiritual life. And only to those who come in the attitude of service will the doors open into the sanctuaries of

[2] *The Art of Ministering to the Sick* (New York, Macmillan Co., 1936).

life. Only to them will it be given to see into the true inwardness of human nature. Our aim is to train those who serve in the methods of accurate, painstaking, co-operative observation and interpretation which will enable us through long-continued effort on the part of many workers to arrive at a true understanding of the laws of the inner life.

The basis upon which I have been able to bring theological students to the hospital has been that of performing some simple service the value of which would be generally recognized by the hospital community and which would at the same time give them an opportunity to study the behavior of our patients. This involved an alteration of my original understanding with the superintendent. At the time I accepted the chaplaincy at Worcester it had been agreed that I was not to be a recreational officer. My task was to conduct the religious services, to get acquainted with the patients, and to give them such personal help and comfort as I could. I was also to be allowed to attend staff meetings and to do intensive work with certain types of cases. With the adoption of the plan for giving clinical experience to theological students I became interested in other kinds of service. I did not propose to bring in novices and turn them loose on the wards to do religious or therapeutic work.

The necessary opportunity I found first of all in the work on the wards. My own experience as a patient had convinced me of the importance of that work. I had myself had the experience of being severely beaten up without provocation by some young attendants and I knew very well that even in the best hospitals, in spite of all the precautions taken, there would be found much of such brutality. I had also known how much it meant to have the right sort of attendants. I had thus become convinced that there is probably no one in the employ of the hospital upon whom the welfare of the patient is more dependent than the nurse or attendant who is with him all day long. But to secure the right sort of attendant was no easy matter in those days before the depression. The limitation in pay and the fact that the position carried with it no promise of a career and no encouragement to homemaking made the situation difficult to rectify. There were indeed devoted men and women whose faithful and unostentatious service on the wards cannot be too gratefully recognized, but the fact remains that in the pre-depression period the new male attendant, as revealed by a study at Worcester, was a man with a mental age of about thirteen years who had no interest in his patients or in the problems which they represented. He was generally a floater who had previously worked in some other hospital, who stayed about three and a half months and was then discharged for inefficient service or brutality or drunkenness, or else he would leave without notice. This situation has been greatly changed since the depression. The turnover is now much less and it is easier to secure good men. But in 1925 it was otherwise and the hospital was quite ready to make use of some intelligent and willing college graduates who were keenly interested in the patients and their problems. These men were placed on the admission wards where they had an opportunity to deal with all kinds of cases. From the standpoint of the student this work on the wards has the advantage of bringing him into close contact with the patients. He sees them day in and day out. He is able to observe what they do with their leisure time, what attitude they take toward their work and toward other people and how they meet the irritations, disappointments, successes, setbacks, and other critical situations which because they are genuine furnish the really reliable tests of character. He has also plenty of chances to hear the patients tell of their experiences and to draw them out a bit. He has thus an excellent opportunity to obtain an insight into the mind of the patient. In order to take advantage of this opportunity a plan was worked out for observations on the wards, and the notes which our students have turned in have been of real value to the physicians in their efforts to understand the patients' difficulties.

In the beginning these students worked ten hours a day as attendants on the wards. It was found however that after a full day's work there was not much time or strength left over for the reading and case work so essential to their training. We then worked out a plan, which still continues, of pairing the students, each pair being responsible for a full day's work on the ward and also for a certain amount of recreational work for the benefit of the patients. This recreational program included baseball, soft ball, volley ball, bowling, hikes, play festivals, choral singing, home talent entertainments, and the publication, with the aid of mimeograph and bulletin boards, of a news-sheet and of a pictorial featuring hospital scenes and happenings. Throughout, our aim has been to give the patients a chance to do things themselves. By thus reducing the amount of required work and introducing a certain variety into the routine, the student is able to keep fresh and to write up his observations, to do the assigned reading, and to attend the medical staff meetings and the special conferences which are held twice each week for the benefit of the group. In these special conferences the staff members have contributed generously of their time and interest and the student has the great advantage of seeing the same case approached at once from different angles.

While the work on the wards and the recreational program have given our students their footing in the institution, the religious work is the focal point of our efforts both during the summer and during the other nine months.

Both at Worcester and at Elgin I found on my arrival practically the same system — services conducted in rotation by ministers from the city. The sermons were usually long and the devotional service short, the patients being given little opportunity to participate. At Worcester there were no hymnbooks at all for the congregation. The minister and the choir took care of everything, while the people merely sat and listened. At Elgin there were books of the gospel song variety — good of their kind. My first task was to find a book of worship suitable for my purpose. My efforts were however unavailing. I did find at Worcester a hospital hymnal printed by the hospital in 1837. I found also a small book of worship printed by the local Episcopal church for its own evening service. This I found useful. It provided a service in which the people themselves might have a large part not merely in song but also in prayer and response, and the hymns and psalms which it contained, while few in number, were from the literary standpoint excellent. Therapeutically, however, there was much to be desired. Of the fifteen psalms, six were of the imprecatory type. They contained petitions for the punishment of enemies. Certainly my patients did not need to have their persecutory trends reinforced. I was especially struck by the following well-known hymn from the seventh century:

> Christian dost thou see them
>   On the holy ground,
> How the hosts of darkness
>   Compass thee around?
> Christian up and smite them,
>   Counting gain but loss;
> Smite them by the merit
>   Of the holy cross.
>
> Christian dost thou feel them,
>   How they work within,
> Striving, tempting, luring,
>   Goading into sin?
> Christian, never tremble,
>   Never be downcast,
> Smite them, Christ is with thee,
>   Thou shalt win at last.
>
> Christian dost thou hear them,
>   How they speak thee fair?
> " Always fast and vigil?
>   Always watch and prayer? "
> Christian, answer boldly,
>   " While I breathe I pray."
> Peace shall follow battle,
>   Night shall end in day.
>
> " Well I know thy trouble,
>   O my servant true;
> Thou art very weary,
>   I was weary too;
> But that toil shall make thee
>   Some day all mine own, —
> And the end of sorrow
>   Shall be near my throne."

A number of hymns in this little collection did not apply at all to the experiences of my patients, but here was one that did. I am very sure that the writer of that hymn had visited the same infernal regions from which I am trying to rescue my patients, and he had apparently found his way out. At least there is a note of triumph at the end. But would this hymn help? Would it not tend to reinforce the fears and intensify belief in the authority of the hallucinatory processes? It is certainly clear that it not only deals with auditory and visual and tactile hallucinations, but it even calls for action besides. Now, no one can tell me, or anyone else who has visited the wilderness of the lost, that such experiences as that which this hymn describes are not real or that the hosts of darkness are not terrible realities which one is right in fearing. Moreover, I look upon it as sound therapy to help my patients to face the facts, however grim, and yet to remain unafraid because of faith in the Love that has power to cast out fear and overcome evil. Such a hymn has therefore in my judgment real value, but it is strong medicine and must be used with discretion in special cases. It is certainly not for general consumption in a mental hospital.

The questions thus raised led to others and I began an examination of the available hymnals. Among them I found a large proportion of hymns that did not apply to our experiences and needs and not a few which were likely to give suggestions that were definitely unwholesome. I could find none that seemed suited to our requirements. The result was an attempt to supply the needed book myself. I wanted a compact collection of hymns and prayers and passages of scripture, and only those which are likely to bring a message of comfort and hope and courage to those who are traveling through the valley of conflict and shadow. I wanted the book primarily for public worship. It must make possible a service in which the people themselves might have a large part. I wanted it also for personal use. To this end I insisted that the words of the hymns should be printed in full below the music.

In order to make the book practicable for our purpose the cost had to be kept low, for a congregation of patients will not treat hymnbooks any more gently than will an ordinary congregation. This I was enabled to do with the assistance of generous friends who provided a subsidy which covered the cost of setting type and making plates.

This book is now in a second, thoroughly revised edition.[3] There may be some difference of opinion regarding the policy which has guided my selection of materials. I have insisted not only upon therapeutic appropriateness and value, but also upon literary merit and upon theology which does not conflict with present-day knowledge. Material that did not meet these requirements was not included. In the matter of music, Professor Cecil Smith, the musical editor, has sought to bring together a carefully chosen collection of the finest and most singable tunes rather than just the most familiar ones. The fact that many of our hymns were not so well known that established associations between words and tune would interfere favored this purpose. Wherever such associations have been encountered they have been treated with great respect, but we have not hesitated in some cases to replace a difficult or inferior tune by one of outstanding merit and easy range. No gospel songs are included for the reason that I could find none that met the requirements.

For our own use the book has proved most satisfactory, more so than I had anticipated. I knew that in the Middle West the gospel songs are dear to the hearts of Protestant people and at the time I came to Elgin I was informed by those in charge of music at the hospital that the patients would not sing anything but a limited number of gospel songs. This has however not proved to be the case. Many of our people here have been accustomed to good hymns. We have also had the help of a patients' choir organized and trained by our students.

This choir has proved to be a most interesting project and I am more and more impressed by its therapeutic value. Among the 4500 patients in this hospital there is not a little real musical talent. Some of our musicians are indeed not very co-operative. Some of them are here precisely because they had become too tempera-

[3] *Hymns of Hope and Courage* (Boston, Congregational Publishing Society, 1932).

mental and difficult to get along with anyone. Some are too far gone to respond to anything. But a considerable number accept eagerly the opportunity to do their bit and have served faithfully and efficiently. Rehearsals are held two and sometimes three times each week. These are looked forward to eagerly by most of the members of the choir and the attendance has averaged about thirty. They seem to get real enjoyment out of these meetings and there seems to be something in the singing together which lifts them out of themselves and their troubles to a higher plane of thought and feeling. The fact that there is a purpose of serving their fellow patients undoubtedly adds to the therapeutic value of membership in the choir. One of our main difficulties as well as one of our chief encouragements is the considerable number of this group who recover sufficiently to go home.

At the religious services the average attendance is about three hundred patients, all of whom come voluntarily. We have an abundance of music and the vested choir is a most important factor. In addition to four congregational hymns we generally have two special numbers, the Gloria, the Versicles and Responses, and a prelude and postlude sometimes with the help of an orchestra. The sermon is generally from ten to fifteen minutes in length. In it we aim to deal with problems which are of real importance to our hearers, such as their adjustment to the locked door, to the requirement of work, to opportunities for play and recreation. We try also to help them to understand the distinction between delusion and belief, between inspiration and hallucination, the danger of seeking alibis or blaming other persons or losing one's way in the land of daydreams. The troublesome conscience, guilt and forgiveness, elation and despair, anger and fear are other subjects which bring a good response, at least, when they are treated in a graphic and interesting way. And this congregation of patients does respond; the way they take part in the service has been for me a continual source of satisfaction.

We have no Sunday school. We do have what we call a mental health conference for a selected group, chiefly of new patients. Here we usually begin with a case taken from some other hospital.

This provides the basis for a discussion which is often both animated and intelligent.

As our project has become more firmly established in the institutional life, it has become possible to do some things which could not be done at first. We are now able to lay more stress upon study and case work on the part of our students, requiring of them less in the way of recreational and ward activity. Our plans for this summer call for intensive study of at least two patients by each man. This study is to include, wherever possible, an investigation of the social background as well as of the patient as we see him in the hospital. In such a study the motive of service is always kept uppermost. The student visits with the patient. He takes him out walking. He is instructed to avoid any lecturing or probing. His task is to be a friend to the patient, at the same time keeping his eyes and ears open, asking questions and responding so as to show his interest and draw the patient out. In addition to increased emphasis upon case study we shall also make more provision for assigned readings and conferences.

In the matter of results obtained through intensive case work I can claim that they have been always on the credit side of the ledger. I can recall no case in which any harm has been done and many cases in which the patient has seemed greatly benefited. This is true of the work done by the students, also of the intensive case work which from the beginning has been part of my own program. I have had a good many irons in the fire and have not been able to give to the case work the prolonged and regular attention which good therapeutic work requires. I have done not a little individual work with patients and have helped to set a number of them on their feet, but it is not possible to tell how far their recovery was due to my own efforts and how far it may have been due to other factors which entered in. Experimentation in the field of psychotherapy is something extremely complex and its results are hard to measure. In the interaction of personalities involved in psychotherapeutic work it is impossible to tell just what factors become operative. A certain intangibility of result is therefore inherent in the problem.

One of our practical problems has of course been that of finances. In the beginning the money we raised through gifts from friends was used in paying our students. This gave rise to a criticism on the part of my medical advisers. They took the position that since the medical interne gets no pay for his period of apprenticeship there was no reason why the theological student should be paid. I was however confronted by certain hard facts. Theological education is today on an entirely different basis from medical education. Where the medical student takes a long and expensive course, paying from three to five hundred dollars a year in tuition in addition to living expenses, the church bears most of the cost of theological education. Few of our theological schools charge tuition. Where they do, that cost is usually covered by scholarship grants. Even the room rent is generally provided for. In addition, at many theological schools provision is made whereby the student can work his way through school, so that it is possible for him to take his entire course and come out in the end free of debt.

Now this may seem a bit like pampering the student, but there is much to be said for it. I am not sure but that it would be a wise policy to have much more of our higher education placed on that basis, with costs defrayed in the case of a rigidly selected group of men. Certainly it seems that a free church unaided by public taxation can hardly recruit and support a married clergy on any other basis. However that may be, the fact remains that such is the system; the summer vacation is a period which the theological student reckons upon to help him pay his way through school, and he usually has opportunities to do remunerative work under the mission boards. To enlist the more promising students I had therefore to meet these conditions; all the more so because the need of clinical experience in the service of the mentally ill is not yet recognized among theological schools. For this reason we offered them attendants' salaries of fifty dollars a month and subsistence. With the adoption of the plan of pairing the men we met the situation by paying every other man out of contributed funds, the hospital paying one man and furnishing maintenance for both. Since the depression it has of course become increasingly difficult to raise money. In consequence what we have raised has been going more and more to pay our supervisors and fellows. The students have received only subsistence except as they have come under some special arrangement, as in the case of scholarship aid granted by their own schools.

The response of the students has been throughout a source of satisfaction. Not only have the number and quality of the applicants increased and improved in spite of the curtailment of pay, but the strongest of those who came have felt so keenly the challenge of this problem that they have shown a gratifying readiness to enlist permanently. That we have not now a larger number of training centers already established has not been due to any lack of able and trained men, but to the slowness of hospital superintendents to recognize the possibilities of such a venture, and the financial obstacles to be overcome.

Of the 160 or more men who through 1933 have had one or more summers of clinical experience with us, five have undertaken the study of medicine, two have gone into psychiatric social work, several are teaching or preparing themselves to teach theology, psychology or sociology. The great majority are either pastors or are preparing themselves for the pastorate. It is to help them and equip them that we are chiefly concerned.

I may say emphatically that we are not encouraging our students to set up as psychotherapists or to start church clinics. We are seeking to help the students, through the study of pathological manifestations, to understand the problems of so-called normal people, and the nature and function of religion in their lives. We insist that the student give his interpretations of the patients whom he is studying in terms of normal reactions, and it is the general testimony of our students that one of the chief values of their hospital experience lies in the light it throws upon their own personal problems. Furthermore, we insist that the student translate the psychiatric terminology into his own vocabulary and learn to recognize the many ancient insights which are today masquerading in new and often barbarous linguistic attire. It is our conviction that effective psychotherapeutic work can be done without any advertising of the fact by anyone who has the necessary understanding and that no one has greater need for such understanding and no one has it in his power to do more effective work in the prevention of mental difficulties than the adequately trained representative of that profession which for centuries has been chiefly concerned with the inner adjustments of men.

Let there be no misunderstanding. We are laboring under no illusion in regard to the adequacy of the present-day understanding of the disorders of the mind or the sufficiency of three months of training, no matter how careful, to place at the disposal of the student the understanding and the tools now available. We recognize that we are as yet but touching the fringes of this most difficult of problems and we have entirely too much respect for the complexities of human nature to suppose for one instant that after one summer at our hospital a student would be equipped to deal successfully with the delicate and baffling inner conflicts of his people. We only hope that we may have been able to start something within him. We hope that we may have kindled in him a new interest in the experiences of living men. We hope that this may lead to a growing insight into the issues of life and death which may be at stake in the lives of even the apparently commonplace, which will pervade and determine his message as a minister and give to it increasingly the authority of truth and the power to inspire conviction. And we hope that he may gain constantly in that understanding and wisdom which will make him for the man in distress a safe counselor and guide. More than this, we hope that this attempt to provide for students of theology clinical experience in the maladies of personality may contribute toward the development of a body of workers who through faithful, co-operative effort over a long period of time may arrive at a new understanding of these disorders of the mind and of the laws and forces involved therein. Such an understanding would, we think, revitalize the enduring elements in the religion of their fathers and lead onward toward the better day that ought to be.

XII

THE DISTINCTIVE TASK OF THE MINISTER
OF RELIGION

AT A RECENT CONFERENCE the leader of a well-known life-adjust-
ment center was asked what he considered to be his distinctive
contribution as a religious worker to the task of personal counseling in which his clinic was engaged. Were there cases which belonged peculiarly to him? Was there some contribution which
he could make beyond that of the psychiatrists and social workers
with whom he was associated? His reply was that he considered
every human problem a religious problem and every effort to help
a brother in need a religious task.

This answer is of interest as a reflection of the groping after new
forms of service and influence which is evident on all sides among
Protestant religious workers and of the inner restlessness and insecurity which it betokens. We see this in such a movement as the
Y.M.C.A., which has grown up alongside of the church and has
devoted itself to a multitude of activities in the effort to develop
" body, mind and spirit." It is to be seen in the development of
the institutional church, in the new emphasis on social service, in
the rural church movement of the pre-war days with its emphasis
upon the economic welfare of the rural family. The present interest in church clinics seems to be very frequently but another manifestation of the same tendency.

The traditional rôle of the minister of religion is revealed by his
characteristic activities. He does certain things which men of
other vocations do not do. He conducts public worship, he

preaches, and he administers the sacraments. Widely as the various church bodies differ among themselves, all of them have the solemn assembly and certain symbolic acts pertaining generally to the major crises of life, such as birth and death and marriage, and to the central religious truths. These are the special province of the priest or minister. Among most church bodies no one but a properly ordained man is authorized to take charge of these. In the matter of sacraments some even go so far as to believe that these operate irrespective of conscious participation either on the part of priest or people. In any case it is clear that the priest or minister of religion in his vocational capacity has always been looked upon as a representative of the superpersonal. He is the servant or agent of God.

This common view of the minister and of his rôle is most important in any consideration of his distinctive task as a personal counselor. In many cases it will be a source of power. In others it will set limits to what he can do. It means that certain types of the distressed will seek him out or welcome his help, and that others will avoid him. It means that to those who do accept his aid he may be able to give a certain service by virtue of that which he represents.

In this inquiry, however, we are not concerned about the traditional views. We are taking nothing for granted. We are recognizing that the explanation of the restlessness which is today so prevalent in liberal Protestantism is to be found precisely in the modern challenge to the assumption which underlies the historic rôle of the minister of religion. We are ourselves scrutinizing those assumptions. Looking at the minister of religion from the standpoint of those who are facing the issues of spiritual life and death and have been thereby cut loose from the moorings of conventional belief, we are asking what insights and what expertness the minister of religion can bring to the problems which they represent. We are inquiring where his help is needed most and where he can spend his time to best advantage.

My own experience may provide the basis for an answer. As chaplain in a mental hospital I recognize my obligation to all the types of sufferers congregated here. It is certainly part of my job to give comfort to the aged and hope to those whose remaining days are likely to be spent within the confines of the institution. I do what I can to give courage and hope to the physically ill and that peace of mind which will favor the curative forces in their operations. The sick and the aged are both likely to be responsive, but in both cases I can do little beyond giving comfort. In the case of the drifter and the crank in their terminal stages I cannot do even that. It would take many, many hours of skilful work to bring about any modification in their attitudes and, with crying need on every side, the time can be used to better advantage. But in the case of those who are grappling desperately with the issues of spiritual life and death, those in whom the better self is struggling for control and survival in the face of unacceptable tendencies which threaten to engulf it, I feel that I have a task that is distinctively my own. In this I am guided not merely by the fact that my own disturbance was of this type, but by the consideration that, if the findings are correct to which this inquiry has led us, such experiences are definitely religious problems. They are clearly related to those through which such men as John Bunyan and George Fox passed in the process of finding themselves. They are also related to those eruptive solutions of inner conflicts which are known as religious conversion experiences. To cases of this type I ought therefore to bring certain insights derived not merely from my personal experience as a patient but from my background as a specialist in religion and from my accumulated experience with other hospital cases. My first task is therefore to discover those persons in whom the better self is really struggling to get possession and in whom the constructive forces have really a chance to win out.

It will thus be seen that in the matter of types of cases, once the physical factors have been ruled out, I would draw the line between my task and that of the physician not so much on the basis of the severity of the disturbance as on the basis of the reaction pattern. I would draw a vertical rather than a horizontal line. Instead of allowing the psychiatrist to remain the exclusive keeper of the lower regions, I am hoping and laboring for the day when the specialists in religion will be able with his help to go down to the depths of the grim abyss after those who are capable of responding, those in whom some better self is seeking to come to birth.

In the matter of techniques there will of course be some differences between those which are applicable to the severe disorders that come to a mental hospital and those which are applicable in the milder disorders. It is harder to establish rapport, and harder as a rule to get our patients to talk of their real difficulties, while their fears, their suspicions, their self-blame generally become so irrational and obsessive as to yield little to treatment. Such techniques as psychoanalysis do not often apply in these cases. The very types that most need treatment of the " surgical " variety, represented in psychoanalysis, are so encased in protective devices as to be impervious. The acute disturbances, with which I am especially concerned, are on the other hand comparable to the breaking open of an abscess. The poisonous matter is already out and no lancing is necessary. What is needed is to give the recuperative forces a chance by restoring the shaken self-confidence and helping the patient to a constructive interpretation of his experience.

Between my own techniques and those of the psychiatrist I recognize no particular difference. I do indeed make use of prayer whenever I believe that the patient wants it or is likely to respond. Wisely used I have found this a powerful instrument in the establishment of rapport with the patient. I also value highly the opportunity afforded me in the religious service. But the form or method of procedure, important though it is, seems to me secondary to the insights which I may be able to bring to the task. What matters most is that I with my particular training and background may be able to see the true meaning of the experience and the fact that my objective is always to assist the better self in its efforts to win out in the face of odds.

In all my efforts I rely upon a simple principle derived from my theological training which seems to me far too little understood.

I refer to the view that *the real evil in mental disorder is not to be found in the conflict but in the sense of isolation or estrangement.* It is the fear and guilt which result from the presence in one's life of that which one is afraid to tell. For this reason I do not consider it necessary to lower the conscience threshold in order to get rid of the conflict. What is needed is forgiveness and restoration to the fellowship of that social something which we call God. In common with psychiatrists generally I therefore try to get the patient to talk, and I am careful never to permit myself to be shocked by any deviations from accepted standards which he may disclose. I then try to *shift the basis of self-respect from the rigid or static type of morality to the dynamic type.* I try to get him to see that no matter how unworthy one may have been he is a good man and worthy of honor in so far as he is earnestly seeking to become better. That, as I understand it, is what Paul meant when he talked about faith as against works and spirit as contrasted with law. I think it is also what my psychoanalytic friends are groping after when they talk about " breaking up the super-ego." I thus try to help the sufferer to get rid of his fears and of his sense of estrangement and to develop a philosophy of life which will enable him to cope with the instinctual drives and bring them into harmony with his ideals. I seek to bring to him that sense of social support which gives peace in the midst of conflict and to reinforce those tendencies which make for progressive unification on a basis conceived as universal and abiding.

The task of the ordinary pastor is, I think, not greatly different. He also will have the sick and the aged and those who are slaves of a situation. In his parish, as our survey has indicated (see pp. 227-28), he finds all the reaction patterns which we find here in the hospital. He merely sees in the more complex incipient forms what we see in the exaggerated and simplified terminal stages. He will have in his group those who are growing in the direction of unification on the basis of the Christian ideal. He will have those who, while professing adherence to the faith of their fathers, have never taken it seriously and have allowed their problems to accumulate. He will have those whose beliefs have suffered some degree of distortion as a means of escaping the sense of personal failure, persons who attempt to maintain their loyalties without paying the price of growth and to this end resort to all sorts of compromises and protective devices. He will have those who make no pretense at conforming to the faith of their fathers and yet are comfortable about it. He will have those who through frank delinquency or mental illness are outside of the pale. And then he will have the distressed — those who, suddenly subjected to the strain of bereavement or of business reverses, are seeking desperately for those values that cannot be taken away; or those who are torn with conflict in the effort to bring the instinctual drives into conformity with the requirements of a new stage of development. In some cases he may have those who are undergoing the stress and turmoil of a mutation process, in whom, as in the case of John Bunyan, some higher possibility is seeking to come to birth.

Toward all of these the pastor will have obligations. The aged, the lonely, the chronic invalid, and those who are carrying on in the face of difficulty will need all the comfort and encouragement which it lies in his power to give. And the group of the faithful, whose recognized leader he is, constitute an invaluable resource. Through them he can greatly multiply his own effectiveness. It must ever be his task to give them the enlightenment and the guidance necessary for their most effective service. And few of them will there be who do not have their own problems and difficulties.

He will also have many dealings with those whose attitudes and values are distorted by unacceptable subconscious desires which they have not been able to bring under control. From our hospital experience he may learn how difficult it is to change such people and how futile it is to reason or argue with them. He may often have reason to wish that they might be consigned to our care. But an understanding of human nature may enable him to get along with them and even to modify their system of beliefs by question and suggestion used skilfully enough to enable them to change without damage to their self-respect.

In the case of those who have rejected the faith of their fathers he will have a problem no less difficult. In their eyes he will have no prestige by virtue of his vocation but rather the reverse. Whatever he accomplishes with this group must be on his own merit, by winning prestige on their terms. It is important for him to understand that standards are commonly functions of the loyalties (see pp. 168–80) and that in the case of those who have rebelled against the primary loyalties and have identified themselves with some group of alien standards, the standards will not be changed apart from personal relationships. The delinquent who has found social support among birds of his own feather and worships at the shrine of Dillinger and Capone can only be changed in so far as he learns to accept another type of hero. It will never be possible to change the attitude of such a person either by force or by reason, but only through the power of admiration and affection. How far it will be worth while for the minister to attempt this will depend largely upon his own qualifications. A distinguished psychoanalyst, when asked what type of cases he would be willing to undertake, replied, " I will take anyone with whom I can establish a transference." This principle applies also to the minister. If he is one who is able to win the respect and the affection of the delinquent and the roughneck or of the social rebel of whatever variety, he can get results. But let him beware of trying to masquerade as a sheep in wolf's clothing. In the case of the delinquent he is certainly not going to raise the boy to a higher level except as he may be able through friendship and understanding to bridge the chasms and win the boy's loyalty in his own true rôle as a representative of society at its best.

Every parish has its own representatives of the down-and-outs. Those who are actually institutionalized are only a fraction of those who might well be. In the parish which we studied the proportion of those sent to institutions as compared with those who might have been was one in four. To the pastor such persons will represent a difficult social problem. It will be for him in many cases an important and delicate task to give help to the families of the unfortunate who have lost out in the struggle and are definitely without the pale. In the case of those who are hopelessly ill mentally, I know of no greater tragedy to the family. It is one far greater than death. And in the case of those who return to the community there is need of a helping hand in order to make possible a new start. In some cases it may be the pastor's task to help rid the minds of the family of the very natural horror at the thought of institutionalizing some loved one who needs it.

But the great opportunity of the pastor is, I think, with the distressed, with those who are in jeopardy, with those who are passing through periods of acute crisis and mutation.

In the case of the bereaved and of the physically ill he may find a readiness to think about the things that really matter, where before other interests and cares had crowded out the ultimate values. At such times he may find a responsiveness which will not be found in other circumstances and, if he have the necessary understanding and delicacy of touch, he may help more than one of these to solve their problems on the level of the religious.

In the case of those who have met with business reverses and economic catastrophe there is likely to be a similar opportunity. In a brief study of the effects of the economic depression upon mental health which I made recently, it was the testimony of all the pastors whom I interviewed that among their parishioners they knew of no cases in which business reverses were clearly primary as a cause of mental ill health. Such reverses served rather to reveal strength or weakness. There were some who simply refused to face the facts, some who whined and pitied themselves, some who became bitter, some who blamed others; there were also those who took the happy-go-lucky attitude; and then there were others, not a few, who came through the period of trial with colors flying. The disappointment and misfortune had merely helped them to see things in true perspective and to find those values which abide. In many of these cases the help of the pastor had been a real factor.

In the case of those who are struggling desperately for self-mastery in the face of unacceptable instinctual claims, the pastor has also a great opportunity and an equally great obligation. It is here moreover that he is today being challenged.

It is probably safe to say that the evangelistic work of the church in the years gone by has centered very largely in this problem of instinctual control. This has not usually been explicit. Generally the language has been veiled and symbolic. Nevertheless the word sin has been rather commonly associated with the idea of sexual transgression. John Bunyan in his autobiography thus makes no mention of any sins except swearing and sabbath-breaking. But it seems clear, as we read the account, that these sins which he does mention are but symbols of those of which he dares not speak. It is equally clear that in this there is no attempt at concealment. He is telling the truth as plainly as he can, but telling it to those who have eyes to see and ears to hear. When Wesley and Edwards and Moody called upon men to repent, we may be sure that while for some that call would mean a summons to come to grips with laziness, or drink, or dishonesty, or hatred and bitterness, it would by most men be interpreted in terms of an unsolved sex problem. Certainly this was true of the Y.M.C.A. evangelism of forty years ago, and the Buchman movement, which is the direct heir of the pre-war Y.M.C.A. evangelism, has made its attack quite openly upon this problem. Not only did the old evangelism attack this problem, but its attitude was rather uncompromising. It had no place in its plan of salvation for any concessions to human frailty except that of marriage and it held over the heads of its adherents the fear of eternal damnation.

This centering upon the problem of sex maladjustment was an inevitable consequence of the fact that for most men, especially in the impressionable adolescent period, this would be the " besetting sin " that was on their minds. It is estimated today that in any group of persons of high school age one in ten will at some time in his life become sufficiently disturbed mentally to warrant commitment to a mental hospital.[1] In the great majority of cases the difficulty will lie in the sexual realm.[2] It was therefore unavoid-

[1] William F. Ogburn, " Frequency and Probability of Insanity," *American Journal of Sociology*, March, 1929.

[2] According to Pierre Janet (in his *Medications Psychologiques*, Paris, F. Alcan, 1919, II, 236) 75 per cent of his cases of mental illness are due to sex maladjustment. Most

able that in the attempt to bring a message of redemption from sin, that message, couched usually in general terms, should be interpreted in terms of release from the sense of guilt due to sexual transgressions.

For this the church is today being severely criticized. It has been justly pointed out that this emphasis on sex maladjustments has served to divert attention from glaring social injustices. It has also been held that the church's teaching regarding sex has been responsible for much unnecessary suffering.

The latter criticism comes especially from medical men. They feel very strongly that only the thorough grounding in the biological and physiological aspects of sex which their training affords can furnish an adequate basis for an intelligent attitude. Religious people without this background have set up standards, they say, without regard to the physiological make-up of men and have so enveloped the subject with fear and mystery and unwholesome prudishness as to induce an exaggerated sense of guilt because of misdemeanors which are trivial and even innocent. Freudian psychology has been particularly severe in its criticisms and under its influence there has sprung up today a growing rebellion against the old taboos. Young people today discuss sex problems with a freedom which would have horrified the previous generation. There is also a tendency to challenge even the most fundamental assumptions of the old sex morality. Such thinkers as Bertrand Russell thus assert that the Christian ideal of marriage without previous sex experience on the part of either husband or wife

---

Freudians explain all functional mental disorder in terms of sex. It is to be noted, however, that they would include in this category all that has to do with the " family romance." Hostility toward the father as the representative of authority is thus taken into account; so also the wish for the death of an overaffectionate mother who stands in the way of the individual's own development. From my contacts with psychoanalysts I get the impression that there is an increasing tendency to give interpretations in terms of the hate motive which is not as yet reflected in the literature. It is recognized that feelings of hostility toward some object of love may be as rigorously repressed and as much a source of the guilt feeling as is erotic craving. Deep depressions, with their characteristic ideas of death, may thus represent self-judgment or self-punishment because of the subconscious desire for the death of a loved one. Hatred and bitterness are of course very pronounced factors in the paranoic reactions.

is a mistaken one and that wherever it is attained the results are generally unfortunate.

This tendency to let down the bars in the matter of extramarital sex relations has of course been greatly furthered by the increasing use of contraceptive devices and prophylactic treatments which permit sex indulgence with practical immunity from the consequences which used to act as deterrents. The result has been a change of attitude and standards on the part of women which as a social phenomenon is symbolized by the spread of the smoking habit among them.

Another trend is that represented by certain physicians who hold that of the two alternatives of extramarital relations and masturbation, the latter is the lesser evil. They therefore seek to get rid of the taboos and advocate a controlled indulgence.

In the claims of medical men to the exclusive control over all that has to do with the problem of sex, liberal clergymen have generally acquiesced. Where forty years ago the Y.M.C.A. presided over this problem in most of our colleges and did most of the personal counseling that was done at that time, we have today the medical expert in the person of the mental hygienist. Throughout the country the old time revivalist has diminishing influence, and among our liberal churches the conversion experience so much in evidence forty years ago is seldom encountered. Most liberal clergymen are inclined to deplore the changes which are taking place in the sex codes, but there are those who accept with enthusiasm the gospel of enlightenment. I think for example of a certain clerical friend of mine who almost every time he sees me is accustomed to bring forth something new in the way of literature on the subject of birth control. Now I am unmarried and that fact is not unknown to him. Neither do I think I have been guilty of showing undue interest in this subject. It is merely that he is a missionary of a new gospel and he has a zeal for making converts.

In trying to find the answer to this most difficult and perplexing problem we may begin by recognizing that technical advice regarding sex adjustments belongs within the province of the physician and not of the minister. I do not mean that there may not be cases, especially in our smaller communities, where friendly counsel on a common-sense basis may not be in order. But it should be clear that the minister is not an expert in such matters and, apart from motivations against which he should be very much on his guard, I can see no reason why he should ever become a colporteur of the contraceptive gospel.

Beyond this point the line is not so clear. In so far as the problem has to do with the philosophy of life and with those loyalties and relationships which are regarded as ultimate, the problem of sex does assuredly fall within the province of the minister.

According to our findings the importance of sex as a factor in mental disorders lies precisely in this realm. We have found no evidence that sexual maladjustment operates directly through its organic effects. It is true that according to Freud there are certain of the neuroses which may be explained in terms of hypertensions resulting from suppression of the impulse, others as psychic weakness due to overindulgence; but the fact remains that one of the outstanding principles insisted on by medical men is that the ill effects of such practices as masturbation are due to psychical rather than physiological factors. They place the blame upon the taboos to which sex is subject and the resulting inhibitions and prudishness, and the sense of secrecy and mystery which prevents its being discussed in good society. Numberless persons therefore have difficulty in making adjustments in the sexual realm simply because they cannot bring themselves to talk over these problems. They are thereby subject to a sense of isolation and of personal failure which according to our findings are at the root of most cases of mental disorder.

From the standpoint of our inquiry it is important to recognize that the taboos, the sense of secrecy and mystery, with which this subject is surrounded, and the sense of guilt attaching to infractions of the accepted sexual code, are social phenomena of profound significance. They are rooted in the biological importance of the sex instinct which has to do with that for which the individual exists, the perpetuation and improvement of the race or species. We live in order that we may pass along the torch of life undimmed and undiminished to oncoming generations. This rule holds for all levels of plant and animal life. The individual lives but for a very short space of time and during his brief existence his vital energies center largely around the breeding and rearing of the young. For this purpose nature makes use of all sorts of marvelous devices and to it the interests of the individual are always subordinated. In mammals, especially in the higher forms, the young are brought into the world at a cost to the mother of pain and even of death. Even in lower forms, like the fishes which spawn and leave the young to shift for themselves, we see such species as the salmon making long and perilous journeys at certain seasons of the year in order that spawning may take place in fresh inland waters where the young may have a chance to live unmolested by their more dangerous enemies. In such species as the bee and the ant, which have a highly developed communal life so specialized that the vast majority of the individuals have no direct part in reproduction, the entire life of the community centers around the queen and the young whom she brings into the world. The community is founded when she takes her nuptial flight. It breaks up when she dies, or else with the appearance of a new queen.

The biological significance of sex is furthermore to be seen in the fact that sexual selection has been the great means of biological adaptation. What a given individual is to be is largely determined with his birth. The new adaptations he will be able to make are relatively limited. The great changes in the introduction of new and better types have been accomplished by the magic wand of breeding, not merely through the intervention of man but by the hand of nature itself.

These same principles apply to man as well as to the lower orders of animal life. There are however certain important differences. There is in man much greater freedom in the matter of sex expression than among the lower animals. Sexual pleasure-taking is not limited to certain mating seasons and today it is becoming more and more divorced from the reproductive function. Man moreover, like the bees and the ants, is a community-forming species with a high degree of specialization, so that it is possible and necessary for many individuals to do their part in the perpetuation and improvement of the race without themselves participating in the reproductive process.

This brief résumé will be sufficient to suggest why the problem of sex figures so prominently in mental disorders and why it is and always will be a religious as well as a biological and medical problem.

It must never be forgotten that religion represents the collective interest. Its function is to conserve the moral achievements which make for the perpetuation and enrichment of racial life. This it does by means of a system of beliefs and attitudes which are accepted by the individual members of the family and are internalized in the form of conscience. The problem of sex therefore figures prominently in every religion and, so far as I am able to discover, no race has ever continued to exist without some form of religion. A religion may thus be looked upon as an attempt to deal with the problem of racial survival and improvement, whose value is to be measured in terms of the results attained.

It must furthermore be recognized that a code of sex morality is properly a subject of social rather than of individual experimentation. Its worth can be determined only by the results secured over a long period of time. One of the dangers which we face today lies in the fact that with sexual pleasure-taking dissociated more and more from the responsibilities of parenthood, we are embarking upon radical experimentation which all too often is guided by individual desires rather than by the collective interest. With the view that there is room for improvement and need for experimentation, no one will disagree. What must be questioned is the likelihood of socially desirable results if the danger signals, set up as a result of ages of experimentation, be disregarded and free rein be given to individual desire. Constructive results are more likely to be obtained under the sort of radicalism represented by Jesus, who insisted that he came not to destroy the law but to fulfill it by transcending it and finding its true meaning.

Professor Hocking has offered what seems to me the right answer.[3] Speaking of those who seek to explain religion in terms of sex, he says that to recognize a relationship between the two is an ancient and true insight. It is however often misunderstood and distorted. Instead of reducing religion to the level of the sexual, a correct understanding requires that the sexual be raised to the level of the religious. With Hosea, with Dante, with Browning we should recognize that sex love at its best approaches religion and only in religion can it find its true realization. What true love wants is union with the idealized other-than-self, which is also what religion wants. Sex love thus seeks not just the finite love object but the infinite, and when it ceases to do so it is no longer love.

One task of the religious teacher today would then be to help his people find the true meaning of the powerful sex urge with which every child of man has to deal. The old " thou shalt nots " are losing their power to restrain. We need not be sorry that they are, provided only that they may have found their fulfillment in a true understanding of the positive values involved.

These positive values are to be found first of all in the home.

This might involve a rediscovery of the sacramental character of marriage. The Roman Catholic church has long had such a doctrine, but by some strange mischance it seems to have missed the real point. For centuries it has taught that the celibate life is the peculiarly holy life, but for those who have not the will nor the self-control necessary to the attainment of this holy life it has provided the institution of marriage. Marriage it has regarded as a sacrament, but the sacrament has consisted in the blessing pronounced by the priest upon a relationship which permits to the individuals concerned the free indulgence of sex desire. True understanding would seem to call for a combination rather than a dissociation of the holy life and marriage. It would set up the ideal of a self-mastery and consecration of will on the part of the individuals concerned which would enable them to practice self-

[3] *Human Nature and Its Re-making* (New Haven, Yale University Press, 1923), chap. 42.

control and to reserve the act of intercourse to such times and such occasions as would have for them a truly sacramental value and serve as the outward and visible symbol of communion, not merely with each other but with God.

It would involve also the recognition that the end of marriage is not romantic love but the bringing into being of new and higher types of personality, the new birth in beauty and power of both body and soul. And that would require the further recognition that in the development of such higher types of personality the home is a factor just as important as the body of the mother, and the social medium is just as potent as the physical.

The insight that sex love at its best is not merely a seeking after the finite love object, but after the Love that is beyond that of father and mother or of husband and wife, has consequences of greatest therapeutic importance. It is a step beyond the Freudian doctrine that no man is well or mature until he has learned to stand on his own feet as an autonomous being. Instead of requiring of us that we should stand " with heads bloody but unbowed under the bludgeonings of fate " as arrogant little captains of our own souls, it provides the basis for a philosophy of life which will enable one to meet outward difficulties and disappointments with something more than stoical resignation. It makes possible the faith that can overcome obstacles and actually change conditions. It is thus at the very heart of the religious message and represents the contribution which is most distinctive of the religious teacher. It is this faith and this alone which has power to bring comfort to the bereaved, hope to the economically crushed, strength to the sick and release to the guilty conscience. It is this insight likewise which alone can transform the loneliness of those whose love has met with disappointment and tragedy.

In dealing with those who are struggling for self-mastery against unacceptable instinctual claims it is therefore first of all important to help them to feel that love and not fear is the one true basis of all ethical codes and that morality, rightly understood, is a matter of inner attitude and purpose rather than of outward conformity. What is needed is to set people free from the paralyzing fears and the sense of condemnation so that they may strive for the attainment of their true objectives. It cannot be too strongly emphasized that it is possible to do this without telling them that masturbation is a trivial matter in which everyone indulges, or without taking the position that it is the normal thing to have recourse to extramarital sex relations. The one thing needful is to release the sufferer from the tyranny of the standardized and to help him to feel that in the eyes of love any man is a good man if he is doing the best he can with the material he has to work with.

Let no one misunderstand. I do not intend to imply that the minister is now to change his tactics and discourse openly on the problem of sex. What I do mean is that he should have a true understanding of what is on the minds of his people and recognize how large a part sex problems play in their lives. I mean that he should be able to interpret the symbols through which they seek partly to express and partly to conceal such difficulties. If he has the necessary understanding he will make it easy for them to talk about their real problems and will thus be in a position to give help where help is needed. I mean furthermore that the minister needs to have faced this problem both in his personal life and in its social significance so that he may be able to give the needed help in a sane and constructive fashion.

This brings us to the last of our groups and the largest, those whom I have called the " unawakened." These are the persons, usually fairly well adjusted in the vocational, social and sexual fields, who have never really come to terms with their ultimate loyalties. They are those who, passively accepting the faith of their fathers, make no determined effort to bring themselves into conformity with its requirements but go through life absorbed all too often in the petty, the trivial, the selfish, and even in that which makes them loathsome in their own eyes. They are thus forgetful of the issues which are of enduring importance to themselves and to the race. I am ready to take the position that it is the church's duty to save such men and to recognize that in order that they may turn and be made whole it may be necessary to disturb their conscience in regard to the quality of the life they are living. And this ought to be done before they perhaps develop symptoms which bring them to some such institution as ours.

If it may seem heretical to my medical friends to speak of the desirability of producing an emotional disturbance, I would make it clear that such disturbances would be only incidental to some needed adjustment. I would remind them that no good physician hesitates to inflict pain in so far as it is necessary to correct some diseased condition, and that he may even produce a lesser disease under controlled conditions in order to avoid a serious disease later on, such as smallpox or typhoid fever. I would furthermore remind them that our findings indicate that the sense of guilt, the self-blame and the emotional disturbances which accompany it are not themselves evils but attempts at a cure. The real evil is the failure to attain the level of adjustment called for in some new period of development and the short-circuiting of the vital energies through easy satisfactions.

Some plan of evangelism must therefore be an essential part of the church's program. No matter how efficient our program of religious education, there will always be those who reach the years of maturity without having attained to the adult level of adjustment. They need to be awakened to the necessity of facing their personal problems while yet there is time. This does not mean that we should go back to an evangelism of the old type. That, as we have seen, has had many shortcomings. It has given treatment without diagnosis. It has applied to all men the same traditional formulae modified only by the insight of the individual evangelist. Sometimes it has been morbidly emotional. Sometimes it has had recourse to questionable techniques in order to add names to the church rolls. The new evangelism must be based upon our growing knowledge of human nature and its problems and it must recognize that the task of reconstruction is merely begun when an individual is awakened to his need. There must in many cases be provision for intensive treatment after the sleeping conscience is aroused and a force of workers equipped to give the needed help. But these differences have to do with methods of procedure and with the clarification of objectives. The essential thing in any effective evangelistic work is the ringing summons to individual men and women to come to terms with their ultimate loyalties.

Would such a summons result again in those conversion experiences which have now so largely disappeared from our liberal churches? That question we cannot answer. We can only say that the new message must be based upon a knowledge of human nature which will enable us to speak no longer as the scribes and interpreters of traditions but with the authority derived from a true understanding of the laws of the spiritual life. We may be sure that such an understanding will never again permit us to have recourse to techniques for working up artificially experiences that are abnormal or to see peculiar value in abnormality as such. We may be equally sure that true understanding will not refuse to recognize true value because it happens to come in ways that are out of the ordinary. We may furthermore be sure that in so far as the evangelistic message is grounded in a vital faith in the actual presence of a Redeeming Love it is likely to be attended with striking manifestations and that new and creative forces will be released.

Upon the problems of religious education this inquiry has no direct bearing. In the mental hospital we have practically no children except for the occasional victim of post-encephalitis or hereditary paresis. Full-blown mental illness seldom occurs before the adolescent period. For this reason no studies have been made of children and their problems. Nevertheless no inquiry into the causation of mental illness can fail to reveal the importance of early training and experience. The insights derived from such an inquiry should therefore have as one of their most important applications a contribution to educational understanding. For this reason, the mental hygiene movement, which grew out of the experiences of the mentally ill, is to be seen centering its attention chiefly upon the problems of child guidance.

It is to be noted that delinquency, in contrast to mental illness, is usually a pre-adolescent manifestation.[4] The delinquent, as

[4] Franz Alexander and William Healy, *Roots of Crime* (New York, Alfred A. Knopf, 1936), p. 278.

we have seen,[5] is commonly an individual who rather early in life has rebelled against the authority of parents and teachers, while the neurotic or psychotic is one who has accepted their authority but has failed in the task of harmonizing the conflicting elements within himself. From the standpoint of inner attitude the delinquent is thus frankly antisocial and is therefore commonly free from inner conflict. The mentally ill is apt to have been the good child, one who is obedient and loyal to those in authority.

The tendency today among mental hygiene experts is to be quite sympathetic with the boy who has rebelled against fussy or arbitrary parental domination. The " mother-fixation " or the " father-fixation " is to them the root of most mental illness and rebellion may therefore be but a necessary stage in development. They are likewise apt to be impressed with the dangers to the individual of overconscientiousness and overreligiousness.

With the view that the growing individual in order to reach maturity must free himself from parental domination our findings are in full accord. I am however inclined to insist that there is only one way in which this can safely take place, that of growth into a more comprehensive understanding and obedience to a higher loyalty. Delinquency, so far as I am able to judge, is very seldom a stage in a satisfactory development and the delinquent is far more a social menace than the psychopathic type. I am therefore convinced that there is another answer to the problem than the one now prevalent. Instead of encouraging rebellion against parental or legal or ecclesiastical authority, it might be well to stress the requirement of obedience to a higher authority. Instead of talking of the danger of too much love between parents and children, we might do well to recognize that true love has always required that the child should outgrow his dependence upon the earthly parents and that it has always been sternly vigilant lest erotic phantasy get mixed up in the relationship. Instead of warning against the dangers of being too good or too religious and advising a healthy sprinkling of wild oats, it might be more true to the facts to emphasize the need of complete commitment to the supreme loyalty and the requirement of perspective to guard

[5] Pp. 144–45, 153, 163, 173, 201.

against the danger of pettiness or morbidness and to allow for the relaxation and recreation essential to efficiency.

The fact that mental disorder very rarely appears until the period of adolescence, suggests the importance of sex maladjustment as a factor and calls attention to the problem of sex education. This inquiry indicates the futility of any sex education which consists merely in imparting information. Information in this field may be productive of harm as well as good. It may merely add fuel to the uncontrollable interests. It may merely increase the mass of terrifying and fascinating material which the boy has been unable to assimilate. What he needs is not just information but a point of view which will make possible a wholesome attitude. He needs to see the problem through the eyes of someone whom he trusts as wise and good, someone with whom he can talk things over so as to socialize and thus assimilate this new field of experience which is involved in the attainment of manhood. As in all psychotherapy it is not what the counselor says to the boy but what the boy says to the counselor which yields the desired results.

The study of the relationship between the adjustments of the parents and those of their children in our small-town parish has suggested the potency of home influences. The fact that the church is characteristically built upon the family as a unit suggests that one of its most important responsibilities and opportunities lies just here. The church school and the instruction which it imparts is much worth while, even though sometimes we get discouraged regarding it; but the important thing is the influence of the church upon the spirit of the home. Its great task is to help the parents to discover Love at its best and to inculcate within their hearts the loyalty to that which is beyond themselves. They will then be prevented from making the mistake of trying to enforce obedience to their own arbitrary commands, a mistake which is sure to develop in the child a moral code based upon fear and upon force. The church's task is to give to the parents a vital faith in the sovereignty of the Love that looks upon the heart rather than upon outward conformity, so that the child may never be afraid to talk over with them his real problems and difficulties and may find encouragement and help toward the attainment of his true objectives.

In this consideration of the task of the minister of religion we have disregarded his rôle as a representative of the superpersonal. We have taken nothing for granted and have considered him rather as one who has devoted himself to a certain realm or aspect of human experience. The priest or minister at his best brings to the task of helping the distressed in mind certain insights. He is versed in the utterances of the great and noble of the race, has traced the adventures of the human spirit both individually and collectively in its quest of the more abundant life. He understands the deep longings of the human heart and the significance of the constructive forces which are manifest alike in the religious conversion experience and in acute mental illness. He recognizes the fundamental need of love, the dark despair of guilt and estrangement from those we love, and the meaning of forgiveness through faith in the Love that rules the universe and in whose eyes no one is condemned who is in the process of becoming better. In such insights lies the important contribution of the competent minister of religion rather than in any particular techniques. Anyone, regardless of his vocation, who has these insights and is able to help the soul in jeopardy to a solution on the level of the abiding and universal is doing the work of the minister of religion.

It would however leave a wrong impression if we did not now point out the conclusion, to which this inquiry has led us, that regardless of the question of metaphysical reality the idea of God stands for an abiding social fact (see p. 176). It represents the love, the fellowship, which has the capacity for universality and without which the individual cannot live. Whether we recognize it or not, we judge ourselves through the eyes of those whom we count most worthy of love and honor, those whose composite impress is represented by our idea of God, and our hearts are restless until they find rest in that fellowship. We may say then that in the society of the future there will ever be a place for the representative of the moral achievements of the race, which need always to be jealously safeguarded, and of the higher potentialities and unrealized possibilities, which are associated with the idea of God. And that representative will in many cases by virtue of his office be able to give help to the individual in distress which otherwise he could not give.

XIII

THE INTERRELATIONSHIP OF INDIVIDUAL
AND SOCIAL SALVATION

IN THAT BEAUTIFUL and moving prayer for personal salvation which is known as the Fifty-first Psalm, we find at the end a brief passage which seems quite unrelated to the rest of the text. After the penitent acknowledgement of his wrongdoing and the plea for inner cleansing and renewal and for restoration of the Holy Spirit, after proceeding to the confident affirmation that the sacrifices of God are a broken spirit and that the broken and the contrite heart will not be despised, the writer exclaims abruptly:

> Do good in thy good pleasure unto Zion:
> Build thou the walls of Jerusalem.

Many critics look upon this passage as a later addition. Whether they are right or not, such a transition from the intimately personal to the social emphasis is quite in accordance with our findings and with religious insight generally.

Throughout the Bible the salvation of the individual seems to be thought of in terms of membership in a group. In the Old Testament we find no thought of any survival of the individual after death. It is the race that survives, the race that is identified with the idea of Jehovah, the God of Abraham and Isaac and Jacob, its forefathers. For this reason highest value is placed upon the integrity of the home. Marital infidelity is an unforgivable sin and childlessness a terrible curse. Leadership is fittingly given not to a succession of chosen individuals, but is hereditary in a royal family. Jehovah himself is often spoken of by the great prophets as the husband of the nation and they represent him as lamenting in words of great beauty and pathos over the unfaithfulness of his beloved. National reverses are interpreted as punishment for national wrongdoing, and some of the prophets venture to predict national misfortunes on the basis of the social injustices which they recognize and to promise protection if the evils are corrected. These prophets are finally forced to the conclusion that only a remnant can survive. The terrible suffering of the Babylonian captivity they interpreted in terms of chastisement for sin, a chastisement borne by the finest and best in the nation on account of and for the sake of the sinful, and they hold forth as the hope of the future the time when their nation should be restored to its old home and redeemed of all its iniquities, and Jehovah their God recognized and obeyed as the God of all mankind.

The salvation offered in the New Testament is likewise in terms of membership in a group, not however a national group but a new and glorified society. If our interpretation of Jesus is correct, his primary conflict was over the problem of racial survival and domination. Forced to the conclusion that the old racial hope of earthly power was not to be realized, he went through a period of agony and suffering equivalent to the experience of personal death and found his way through to faith in a spiritual kingdom. He came therefore preaching that the Kingdom of God was at hand and calling upon the people of his time to seek membership therein. To belong to that Kingdom was of such vital importance that in order to obtain it a man must be willing to give up all that he had, even his earthly life. On the basis of membership in that Kingdom and on that basis alone was salvation to be found; and riches, honor, ethical complacency and all that might induce a false sense of security made salvation very difficult. The Fourth Gospel represents Jesus as using the figure of the vine and the branches to express the view that only through relationship to him could the individual continue to live. In the figure of the human body Paul expresses the same idea. Of that body Christ is the head and the believers are the members. As members of that body they find unity amid diversity and all suffer together and rejoice together. Membership in this body is obtained through baptism, which typifies the experience of dying with Jesus in order to live with him and in him. The concluding vision of the New Testament is that of the holy city, the New Jerusalem coming down from heaven to earth.

Time and again in the cases we have studied we have seen this association of the individual and the social, and we have been led to the conclusion that the problem of the world and that of the individual are closely related. It was, as we have seen, no accident that our peacemaker (see p. 178) through a conflict with an unmanageable sex drive was led to concern himself with the idea of the coming millennium " when all humanity would be striving for one goal and for the kingdom of heaven." Over and over again in those acute conflicts in which the individual in desperation is struggling for the reorganization of his personal life, we see the same concern with the problem of the world and the same transition from the individual to the social which we find in the Fifty-first Psalm. This we have explained as due to the inexorable requirement that each individual must be at one with that which is supreme in his hierarchy of loyalties.

Mental health is not an individual matter. It has to do with our consciousness of right or wrong relationship to those whom we account most worthy of love and honor. The deepest desire of every human heart is that for love. No individual can live for himself alone. He lives for his race and he must be ready if need be to give his life and all that he has for its perpetuation and improvement. This requirement is abundantly in evidence in time of war and upon it the very existence of the race has ever been dependent. The idea of God, which is found at all times and among all races, is a symbol of this collective interest. It originates in the child's experience of complete helplessness and dependence and culminates in the mature in the loyalty which is ready to give itself to the uttermost. It stands for the faith that the love which gives protection and for which one is ready, if need be, to give one's life, is enduring and universal. It is in accordance with this idea of God, under whatever name our philosophy of life permits us to use, that our ethical standards are determined. Through his eyes we judge ourselves. To have that in one's life which cannot be brought before his eyes without condemnation is the essence of what we know as the " sense of guilt " and the source of most mental illness of the functional variety. To be isolated from this deeper self, which is represented by the idea of God, is spiritual death, just as real and just as inevitable as for a cell to be cut off from the organism to which it belongs.

It follows therefore that no consideration of problems of mental health is possible apart from their social ramifications. These problems can be understood only in the light of the loyalty to which the individual is committed or that which he is seeking to evade. They can be understood only as we consider what kind of society he wants to create and perpetuate and be identified with. Personal salvation can be found only in reconciliation with this deeper social self and in commitment to the task of transforming the personal and social life. This involves the attempt to establish some sort of utopia. Without some such objective there can be no growth and no progress. Without it the destructive, individualistic forces take the reins and the group or the nation disintegrates.

Religion is thus inherently social as well as personal. It is rooted in a loyalty that is looked upon as so important that for it the individual is ready to live and, if necessary, to die. Its task is to perpetuate the moral achievements by internalizing in ever widening circles and in successive generations the loyalties to which it is committed and the moral ideal toward which it strives to grow.

It is of course true that religion in practice fails tragically to enlarge its vision and falls short of its ideal. This failure is due to weaknesses and limitations inherent in human nature. Both in its strength and in its weakness we may distinguish certain chief types of religion.

The commonest type is that which may be designated as " tribal " religion. This is the religion in which the primary loyalties remain paramount. It is the religion which is taken over from the parents and early guides and is never thoroughly assimilated or transcended. It thus remains something rather superficial, a set of beliefs and attitudes taken over on the authority of others and never really incorporated into the philosophy of life of those who profess them. It is the religion of those who would maintain their loyalty and find salvation without paying the price necessary for growth and achievement. It is to be seen in those persons, usually fairly well adjusted as regards that which is contemporary and local, who go their way without taking much thought concerning the true end and meaning of their lives until perhaps some period of crisis comes. It is seen also in those whose religion is confined chiefly to ceremonials on such occasions as death and birth and marriage. It is the religion of ecclesiasticism, or ceremonialism, of nationalism. Its virtues are generally not those which pertain to the weightier matters of the law; its loyalties are sectarian and partial, not universal in their outlook. By giving support to minor loyalties it undergirds strife and conflict and makes the war danger more terrible.

Against the type of religion which spent itself in the observance of new moons and fasts and in the offering of sacrifices the old Hebrew prophets had constantly to fight. Jesus clashed with it and thereby met his death. All down through the ages those who have attained to the broader vision and the more comprehensive understanding have had this tendency to reckon with.

Among those who have achieved some degree of emancipation and first-hand vision we may distinguish two chief types, each with its own points of strength and weakness.

We have in the first place those who have enlarged their horizon by turning their attention outward. This group is very much in evidence in this day and age when the telescope and microscope have extended the universe beyond the power of the human imagination to grasp. This type we see in the scientist and the reformer who in their devotion to truth or to a cause find the end and meaning of their lives and something corresponding to religion. The weakness of such a religion, from the standpoint of our inquiry, lies in its tendency toward depersonalization and in the fact that it is largely limited to those who have Ph.D. degrees. It may bring emancipation but it brings little of that comfort and social support which the human heart requires. All too often, moreover, the scientist loses sight of human values. Even in the study of human society he may become so absorbed in things statistical or institutional that he may forget that society is made up of persons and that it is only as we are able to see the institution or the social situation in the light of personal experience that we shall be able to attain any measure of true understanding. Worst of all, he may become so engrossed by his special problems that he fails to see those special problems in their larger setting. He thus loses his sense of perspective and of reverence. He is then apt to develop that dogmatism and cocksureness which indicate that one is out of right relationship with the universe. The reformer likewise, in his zeal for improving conditions, too often forgets that increased production and better housing, or whatever it may be, are not ends in themselves but are important only in so far as they contribute to the enrichment of human life.

Finally we have the type with which this inquiry is more particularly concerned, those who in some searching experience have been brought face to face with the ultimate realities of life and have reorganized their lives on the basis of a " mystical " experience. The old Hebrew prophets belonged in this group; so also did the saints of the Middle Ages. Representatives of this type we may see in those sects which lay stress upon the experiences of conversion or illumination or sanctification. Such experiences serve in many instances to enlarge the horizon, to bring new insights and release new sources of power. Their great importance lies in the fact that the individual is brought into that fellowship which has the capacity for universality, that which is represented by his idea of God. All too often, however, the individual who passes through such experiences, especially experiences of the more searching type, does not succeed in effecting a satisfactory integration with the external world. His attention may remain centered in the inner world and even where he may get a following or identify himself with a group his outlook may remain circumscribed. All too often the fellowship into which he enters remains limited to his own type and the divine is for him not greatly above his own level. Under such conditions the energy which is released is applied in ways that have limited social value. Such religion may serve to enable such persons to live and function in the world of men but it is the religion of a limited group. It may found convents or save particular types of souls but without the larger outlook it cannot contribute much to the redemption of mankind.

Common to all these types is the constant social reference. There is the effort to fulfill the requirements of loyalty to that which is accounted best in social experience. The average man may seek to fulfill that requirement at the lowest possible cost but those loyalties must be maintained. The scientist and reformer maintain them in the larger outlook and in devotion to truth and to a cause. The mystic feels that he has attained to fellowship with an eternal Love. Personal salvation is thus found only in the identification with some Greater-than-self. Social salvation will be achieved only as this Greater-than-self can become an object of devotion so universal that all men will be bound together in the bonds of a common loyalty which will have priority over the claims of family and clan and nation.

It follows therefore that salvation, both individual and social, is to be found by entering into that fellowship which has the capacity for universality. To be cut off from this is, as we have seen, the root evil in mental disorders of the functional type, something which brings to the individual isolation and death and destruction. To fall short of it and devote one's self to some lesser loyalty is the cause of most of our social evil and distress. To attain to it means the peace and joy and stability of character that cannot be taken away because it rests on that which outward vicissitude and even death cannot destroy. Such salvation through the fellowship of the spirit is open to anyone, no matter how imperfect, who is ready to acknowledge and renounce that which has been separating him from this fellowship and to give himself earnestly to the pursuit of the better life. Herein lies the meaning of Paul's doctrine of justification by faith. Salvation is for him not a matter of doing things. It is neither a matter of ethical correctness nor of service to one's fellows. It is a matter of inner attitude and spirit, a living relationship with the fellowship which is united by its common loyalty to Jesus Christ and its common struggle for the better personal and social life.

And the significance of Jesus may be found in the fact that in him we see a combination of these three types or tendencies at . their best. According to our interpretation he was a patriot to whom the welfare of his people was as his own personal welfare. He was a man of vision and understanding, keenly interested in the life around him and able to penetrate straight to the heart of things. He was able to reduce the complex entanglements of tradition and legalism to the simple principle of love to God and to one's neighbor and able also to deal so honestly and intelligently with the facts as to arrive at the conclusion that the wishful thinking of his people was not to be realized. It was this conviction apparently that carried him through an experience equivalent to personal death. From this he emerged with new insights and with a profound sense of fellowship with the God of his fathers which he was able so to synthesize with the external world that his life and teaching have furnished inspiration and guidance to multitudes of the finest spirits throughout the past nineteen centuries and even to the present day.

IN CONCLUSION

As we now approach the end of this book, my mind goes back to the beginning of my journey into the lower regions. Once more I am standing on the threshold of the limitless unknown, face to face with death and life. It is not merely my personal fate that is at stake. I see unfolding before me the great drama of the ages. Amid all the interplay of forces and against the dark background of the selfish and the cruel and the lustful, I see continually manifesting itself a great and loving Spirit, at work in the homely aspirations and loyalties of ordinary folk as well as in the heroic endeavors of prophet and leader. Step by step, through infinite toil and sacrifice and hard-won victory, mankind has been going forward to new and higher levels and a richer and more complex life. But now everything is in the balance and God himself is in peril. Our Christian civilization is in jeopardy and the world is likely to lapse back into barbarism with the cruel, the selfish and lustful forces in full control. Once more there comes over me the realization of how little this life of mine counts except as I am able in some small measure to contribute to this plan of the ages. Once more I am concerned less about myself than about those without whom life is valueless to me. All this I see not as a mere intellectual proposition. I feel it as a grim and awful reality. It is brought back to me with particular vividness in the Statement of Belief which marks the transition to the definitely abnormal condition. This Statement of Belief may serve to suggest the central thesis to which we have been led by this inquiry. It also sounds the note with which I would bring this book to a close. I therefore quote it in part:

I believe in the Love which came to my rescue on that Easter morning long years ago, the Love that has pitied my weakness and borne with my failures and forgiven my sins, which has lighted the way through the dark nights of despair and has guided me through the awful wilderness of the insane where the going is difficult and very dangerous. I believe that this Love is one with the God who through all ages and among all races has sought to make himself known to the children of men.

I believe that this God was once perfectly revealed in the life and character and teachings of Jesus of Nazareth. His patience with our shortcomings, his compassion upon our infirmities, his unfaltering faith in men, even in his enemies, and his method of dealing with them, not through force but through the power of love, culminating in his death upon the cross, where he died, the just for the unjust, the perfect for the imperfect, the strong for the weak.

(At this point the abnormal condition began.)

And this process has been going on for nineteen centuries. The strong have been giving themselves for the weak and the perfect for the imperfect. Thus a crossing process has resulted. The divine has in consequence been coming into the world disguised in ugliness, crippled by disease, shackled by sin, and impotent with weakness.

I believe that the weak and the imperfect should no longer accept this sacrifice, but that they should be willing now to give their lives, the imperfect for the perfect, the weak for the strong, that the divine may be freed from its prison-house of deformity and may be able to come into the world in beauty and power and not in disguise. Then may the reign of love replace that of brute force and ruthless competition, where survival goes to the strong and to the merciless. And even as the divine has pitied our weakness and loved us in our imperfections, the weak and the imperfect should take pity on his suffering and impotence.

It will be noted that the first part, while written under strong emotion, follows more or less conventional lines. It came as the result of considerable reflection and had been worked over several times. At the point where the definitely abnormal condition begins, there came a sudden invasion of something quite foreign to all my previous thinking and reading. It came surging in as from an outside source and I wrote down what came to me just as rapidly as I could write, feeling myself merely a passive instrument. Ideas followed each other in rapid succession, ideas that were strange and terrifying and utterly unheard of. These ideas carried conviction with them. They had to do with that which was beyond the range of normal vision and they shattered completely the foundations of my accepted system of beliefs.

The nature of that experience of mine has, I think, been somewhat clarified through this inquiry. It has been shown that it does not stand alone but belongs to a group of experiences which are characterized by the same general constellation of ideas. It has been shown that these experiences are essentially purposive. They are attempts to solve difficult personal problems and tend either to make or break. Among the hospital cases we have found a large proportion of the acutely disturbed who went to the back wards as hopeless wrecks. We have found others, not a few, who emerged from these experiences freed from malignant sets and attitudes and with their problems largely solved. We have found that these acute disturbances which can be observed in any mental hospital bear a striking resemblance to certain types of religious experience. This experience of mine, mental disorder of the most profound and unmistakable variety, was yet for me religious experience in that it brought with it a correct solution of a very difficult personal problem, the solution which is embodied in this Statement of Belief. It was a solution which came automatically through the spontaneous resolution of the subconscious elements that were present, just as previously all my major decisions had been made automatically, although without any such profound upheaval.

Our inquiry has shown furthermore that back of the more constructive solutions resulting from these acute upheavals is a common basic experience. In my own case the basis of the solution lay in the giving up of a hope on which I had staked everything, so that to give it up was for me as the giving up of life itself. So far as I have been able to determine, some renunciation equivalent to the experience of death is characteristic of other acute upheavals. Such experiences may then be looked upon as attempts, sometimes more and sometimes less successful, to eliminate that which is blocking development and preventing the achievement of some higher level of adjustment. They would thus be attempts to carry through the principle enunciated by Jesus of losing one's life in order to find it, of giving up some lesser good or some conflicting desire in order to make possible an integration on the basis of loyalties and values which are regarded as supreme. It is apparently for this reason that nearly always in such experiences there is the sense of being identified with some great superpersonal Being. Those who pass through such experiences may and usually do feel their own infinite littleness. At the same time they also feel themselves one with God or with Christ or with whatever other symbol of the collective they may have chosen. And standing on the threshold of the mysterious and limitless unknown, face to face with the stern realities of death and life, they become profoundly concerned over the fate of the group or race.

Such ideas are to be found in case after case not only among our hospital patients but in some who are accounted among the great religious geniuses of all time. We have thus been led to the conclusion that the distinction between the eruptive solutions of inner conflicts such as we see in George Fox and Saul of Tarsus on the one hand and those which we find in such large numbers on our hospital wards is to be drawn solely in terms of the results achieved. Such results are moreover largely predetermined by the character elements which the individual brings to the crisis experience. Regardless of outcome, we have found marked religious concern characteristic of acute disturbance and involving a sense of union with the Greater-than-self which places such experiences definitely in the mystical group. There is thus a definite relationship between the mystical and the pathological which is to be explained by the fact brought out in this study that religious concern is invariably associated with the attempt to grapple with the vital issues of life. And wherever the conflict is keenest, there we are likely to find both religious and pathological manifestations.

In accordance with scientific procedure, which I have throughout sought to follow, I have been trying to discover relationships within experiences which any qualified investigator may observe and to make no claims beyond those which he should be able to verify and accept. Conclusions that cannot be verified by others I have tried to avoid and I have sought to use terms which would be intelligible and acceptable to workers who had not, like myself, visited the wilderness of the lost and who could not therefore share the beliefs based particularly upon that experience. I have thus, as a rule, avoided the word " God." I have referred instead to the " Greater-than-self," to " that which is supreme in our hierarchy of loyalties," to the " symbol of the collective " or to " the composite impress of those we count most worthy of love and honor." Such terms are neutral. They point to social facts which no competent and fair-minded man can deny and they suggest certain significant relationships. But I should not be telling all the truth if in bringing this report to a close I did not recognize the inadequacy of that which is objective and verifiable and if I did not bear witness to the conviction based upon an experience which cannot be repeated under controlled conditions, a conviction which no consideration of the facts permits me to escape, that back of this solution of my problem there was something more than just myself, something not just blindly purposive but a guiding Intelligence. There is always a tendency for the vivid sense of reality to pass as these experiences recede into the distance. The real danger is, I think, that of forgetting and of failing to heed the vision that comes to us at those times when we stand face to face with the ultimate realities of our lives. It would be indeed a tragedy in my own case if the idea of God did not remain for me something very much more than just a symbol.

I feel it in order also to add that my concern over the world situation has not passed with the solution of my own personal problem. I still feel that the fair civilization which owes so much to the life and teaching of Jesus of Nazareth is standing today in greatest peril. After a century of unparalleled development during which the human race found itself with undreamed-of power in its hands, a century during which hope ran high for the coming of a new and better social order, the forces of evil seem in the ascendant and the tools and the resources which ought to be used for the advancement of human welfare are potentially instruments of destruction. We are living in a sick and suffering world and the terror and agony of those dark days in the lower regions are still present in the black and threatening clouds which lower above us. The god of war and hatred, of suspicion and greed, seems likely once again, in the name of the lesser loyalties, to conscript the lives of men and to use up their latent heroism for mutual destruction.

Against this dark background the guiding Intelligence whose hand I see in the solution of my personal problem remains for me one with the universal Love at the heart of all humanity who through all ages and among all races has sought to make himself known to the children of men. I still see that Love most perfectly revealed in the life and character of Jesus of Nazareth, especially in his death upon the cross. That death upon the cross represents to me the Love which is ready to give itself to the uttermost for the imperfect and the erring, a Love that respects the integrity of each individual and refuses to coerce or to require obedience to the end that all may be bound together not through fear and through force but by the free response of love.

And standing once again in retrospect upon the threshold of that inner world of the ultimately real there comes once more the summons to learn the lesson of the cross. That summons calls upon us to abandon all those subterfuges which for so many centuries have permitted frail humanity to evade its clear meaning. Instead of the historic doctrine of the vicarious atonement, it calls upon us to see in the death of Jesus the way of life. It bids us see in it a challenge to that complete commitment to the God in whom he believed and to the cause which he represents. Such commitment is the one true response to the love represented in Jesus and in those who have shared his spirit. It is also the one way to personal and social salvation. Thus only can we escape from the tyranny of the standardized and from the domain of fear and of force into the glorious liberty which the Apostle Paul proclaimed, the liberty of those who, no matter how weak and imperfect, have entered into the universal fellowship which is engaged in the age-old struggle for the redemption of the world and have found thus peace and joy even in the midst of conflict.

TECHNICAL TERMS AND CONCEPTS

TECHNICAL TERMS AND CONCEPTS

IN ACCORDANCE with the methodology adopted in this inquiry we have begun with the raw material of human experience and have allowed definitions to wait upon a more adequate knowledge. I have looked upon exactness of definition as dependent upon the formulation of conclusions and generalizations. These I have sought to work out empirically. I have therefore been content to make use of terms current in the fields we have been exploring. This plan has offered some difficulties in that the fields under consideration are divided between two professional groups, each with its own vocabulary and neither one knowing much about the other. Now that we have come to the end of this inquiry it may be an aid to clarification if we attempt to define some of the more important terms and concepts which we have been using. This is the more necessary for the reason that so far as possible I have been giving preference to the less technical terms. It is inevitable that such terms, which are employed loosely in the common usage, should have taken on for us somewhat special meanings and that even the technical terms will in many cases have been modified in order to incorporate the new insights derived from this inquiry.

From the General Field

PERSONALITY. The total make-up of the individual with special reference to the distinctive features as contrasted with those that are common to the group. It includes the temperamental and intellectual traits as well as that integration of belief, attitude and action which constitutes CHARAC-TER. The latter is personality viewed from the standpoint of morality. The term SELF is personality viewed from within.

We have taken the view that personality develops much as the body develops through the incorporation of new materials (experiences) into an existing organization through the use of language (see pp. 151–52).

CONSCIOUSNESS. The awareness or perception of meanings which makes possible the assimilation of new experiences. I have followed Dewey in recognizing no sharp cleavage between the field of clear awareness and the background of dim awareness. I have therefore given preference to the term " subconscious " as against the Freudian concept of the " unconscious." According to Dewey the mind is an organized system of meanings, a great background and foreground which is implicit and operative in any conscious state or thought. Sensations he regards as calls to action on the part of the entire organism and consciousness is analogous to a searchlight which plays upon those spots where adaptations have to be made and action taken. Mind is thus contextual, persistent, a constant luminosity, while consciousness is a bright light which is focal and intermittent (*Experience and Nature,* pp. 298–303). Once the adaptation has been made and the new experience incorporated through the discovery of its meaning, it tends to sink back into the realm of dim awareness, there to function automatically or to lie dormant until called out by some appropriate stimulus (see pp. 151–52).

PHILOSOPHY OF LIFE. A term which denotes personality as viewed from the standpoint of meanings. It corresponds to the German term *Weltanschauung* and signifies the individual's orientation with reference to the external world, his conception of himself and of his purpose in life, his hierarchy of loyalties and values and his system of beliefs and attitudes. The development of such a system of meanings is dependent upon the use of language. This means that it is a social process. It involves the incorporation within the individual of the group organization and system of meanings. While thus growing out of clear awareness, and depending for its framework upon that which can be put into words, the philosophy of life is to be thought of as something vastly more than that which is clearly articulate. It is the entire system of meanings which influences and determines all his reactions and all his thinking. It may even include much that has never been put into words but which as feeling or intuition constitutes a sort of fringe to the clearly conscious and has an important directive influence (cf. Dewey, *Experience and Nature,* p. 299).

DESIRE. A term used to denote the awareness, whether clear or vague, of an unsatisfied need. Throughout this inquiry the dynamic basis of the personality has been assumed and interpretations have been given in terms of the desires and needs. While thus recognizing some sort of vital urge, some instinctual drive or drives as back of all the manifestations of human life, our findings lead us to look upon the perception of meanings as the organizing principle. We have found the cause of functional mental disorder in the presence of desires which are unacceptable to the social self and we have explained the remarkable distortion of belief in the paranoic as the attempt to incorporate or assimilate the disowned desires. Our inquiry has thus led us to look upon the social or " integrative " desires for *response* and *recognition* as representing the fundamental need of every individual. We have also been led to distinguish the " segmental " desires which by their partial and regressive character tend to conflict with the requirements of the organized self (pp. 149–52, 156–57, 172–75).

AFFECT. A technical term used to denote the pleasure-pain elements in the response to a stimulus. It is thus to be distinguished from the motor and from the cognitive aspects of the response. The affective elements in the response range in intensity from APATHY (absence of affect) to the exaggerated responsiveness to the external world which we find in " manic " states and the profound inner turmoil of the catatonic upheavals. They differ also in kind or quality, as in joy, sorrow, bitterness, etc. The term EMOTION, which is frequently used as a synonym, is also frequently used to denote the total immediate response in contradistinction from the rational response which characterizes volition. The term FEELING, which in common speech is likewise used interchangeably with both " affect " and " emotion," denotes also a nonverbalized awareness which is more or less synonymous with INTUITION.

ATTITUDE. The emotional " set " which predisposes the individual to respond in a particular way to certain stimuli. The attitudes may be thought of as the motor and affective aspects of the individual's organized experience or philosophy of life.

SOCIALIZATION. The term " socialization " we have used to denote the identification of the individual with his group. We have been led to the view that man is a social being. He must be able to feel himself a functioning part of some social whole, for the sake of which he can, if necessary, even give his life. The value judgments of the individual are thus dependent upon his social relationships. He judges himself, his possessions, his accomplishments through the eyes of those with whom he seeks to be identified and to feel himself " isolated " from them is, according to our findings, the root evil in functional mental illness (cf. pp. 172–80). We have seen that socialization may take place on different levels, from that which is conceived as universal and abiding, as in religion at its best, to the acceptance of the ideals and the finding of satisfaction in the approval of a criminal gang.

ISOLATION. A term used in this book to denote an inner attitude or state of mind characterized by the sense of estrangement from those with whom the individual seeks identification. We have explained it as due to the presence within the individual of instinctual tendencies out of harmony with the fellowship to which he aspires and which he is unable either to renounce or control or to acknowledge without fear of condemnation (p. 144).

LOYALTY. Used in this book in the special sense of an accepted identification with some person or group. The term " primary loyalty " is used to denote the relationship toward the parents and early guides with its mingled attitudes of obligation, fear and affection. The term " ultimate loyalty " is used to denote the identification with the social whole which generally is symbolized by the idea of God. The relationships toward those who are looked upon as representatives of authority differ widely in the relative strength of fear and obligation as compared with love and understanding.

CONSCIENCE. We have followed Professor Hocking in regarding conscience as an awareness of success or failure in maintaining one's status and one's growth. It interposes a check when any act is proposed which threatens the integrity of the personality. It is also on the growing edge of human nature as a guide in determining the direction of growth (*Human Nature and Its Re-making*, pp. 123–24). Its origin, or basis, we have found in the organized system of meanings and moral judgments taken over from the group, particularly from the early guides (pp. 163–80; also notes to p. 151 and p. 171).

CULTURE. A sociological term denoting the system of attitudes, values and customs held in common by a group of people and relating to their self-maintenance and self-perpetuation. It follows from our findings that culture, as thus defined, is dependent upon a common loyalty. With the acceptance of that loyalty by the individual members of the group, the system of values and attitudes which the group holds is internalized in the form of conscience. The curbing of the antisocial tendencies is thus provided for not through force from without but through individual self-discipline.

RELIGION. Socialization on the level of that which is conceived as universal and abiding. It involves the sense of identification with a fellowship which has the capacity for universality. This may or may not include the idea of God. Usually it does. It involves also certain behavior sequences. According to our findings an acutely disturbed patient, struggling for survival against forces which threaten to engulf him, is likely to be preoccupied with the problem of his own relationship to God (pp. 48–53). In so far as he has the sense of mystical identification and in so far as his conduct is in keeping with his ideation, he is regarded as religious, no matter how grotesque his ideas and no matter what the outcome may be. And to the extent that he succeeds in achieving a unification of personality on the basis of what for him is the supreme loyalty, to that extent we have recognized the experience as religious, regardless of its social acceptance. We must then distinguish between superior and inferior types of religion. The superior type would be that which makes for unification with the finest potentialities of the human race.

Our findings indicate that religious concern is associated with the attempt to face the facts of the life situation in the light of ultimate loyalties and values. It does not tend to appear in the reactions of drifting and of concealment (pp. 48–53, 79–82, 212–15).

From the social standpoint religion is the attempt to establish and perpetuate some common loyalty and the moral achievements and insights associated with it. Organized religion centers in a common loyalty and in the purpose of fostering the potentialities which it represents (pp. 204–5).

From the Field of the Theologian

THEOLOGY.   The attempt, either individually or collectively, to organize and scrutinize the beliefs regarding the end and meaning of life, the spiritual forces which operate within us and the relationships which exist between their various manifestations, all in the light of the belief in a supreme reality to which men generally give the name of " God."

From ethics and philosophy it is distinguished by the fact that it is concerned with the realm of religious experience and belief; whereas ethics is concerned with interpersonal relationships and values without reference to the faith in a superpersonal Being and philosophy is the attempt to organize and interpret all of human experience.   As currently used in our schools the term " theology " is limited to the consideration of the fundamental tenets of the Christian religion as represented in the authoritative sources. In this inquiry we have been concerned with the religious beliefs of a number of individuals, most of whom have been reared in the Christian faith. We have sought to determine the origin and meaning of these beliefs, their function in the individual's life, and their implications for a general system of values.

PRIEST.   According to anthropologists no race of men is known which has not had some form of religion and generally a group of men set apart as custodians of that religion.   For such custodians of the racial heritage the generic term is " priest."   The ancient Hebrews, in addition to the priests, had a class known as " prophets."   The latter represented the more spontaneous manifestations of religion, while the priests were those who were trained in the traditions and ceremonies.   The term " minister," which is used in this book, is current among Protestant churches.   It had originally rather the prophetic connotation but has today elements of both.   The priestly class in the earlier stages of civilization has been the custodian not merely of religion but also of education, medicine and science.

MYSTICISM.   Religion shows two common tendencies.   It may place the emphasis upon form, ceremony, custom, tradition; or it may stress experiences which are interpreted as manifestations of the superpersonal.   The latter is what is meant in this book by the term " mysticism."   A mystical experience is one which brings to the individual a sense of fellowship with God.   According to Professor Coe the distinguishing characteristic and the primitive root of the mystical is to be found in automatic experiences interpreted as possession (pp. 92–93; also 30 ff., 79–82 and 191–92).

GOD. According to our findings the idea of God, regardless of the metaphysical reality which may or may not be involved, stands for a social and psychological fact of basic importance. It symbolizes that in the individual's social experience which he counts of highest value and with which he would be identified. It represents the composite impress of those whom he counts most worthy of love and honor (pp. 177, 195–201). It is likewise the symbol of the abiding collective interests (pp. 286–89).

SIN. A tendency or an action which is out of harmony with the fellowship to which the individual aspires or ought to aspire and with the level of development to which he ought to attain (pp. 201–10). It is more specifically a breach of trust as regards what he conceives to be his ultimate loyalty (p. 209).

GUILT. A legal term which is used interchangeably with the term "sin." It is current today in psychiatric circles, while the term "sin" is frowned upon.

It is important to distinguish between the *sense of sin* or *guilt* and the *actual faultiness* or "state of depravity" which is at variance with the requirements of the highest fellowship and of which the individual may be unaware. The sense of sin denotes the awareness of something within which would be condemned by those with whom he seeks identification and which, so long as it is not brought out into the open and dealt with correctly, will separate him from their fellowship. The consciousness of sin, according to Christian theology, is the first step in the process of salvation.

For a consideration of the various ways of dealing with unacceptable tendencies see pp. 142–62; also 201–10.

CONVERSION. The more or less sudden change of character from sinfulness to righteousness or from indifference to spiritual awakening which, ever since the time of John the Baptist and Saul of Tarsus, has been recognized and cultivated in the Christian church (pp. 90–93, 158–59, 207, 234, 281).

FORGIVENESS. The experience of reconciliation following upon some breach of trust, marked on the one side by the acknowledgement of wrongdoing and the desire to make amends and on the other side by the capacity to understand and the willingness to resume friendly relations.

SALVATION. The release from the sense of isolation and the restoration to fellowship with God (mental health) which follows immediately upon the experience of forgiveness (pp. 210–11).

SANCTIFICATION. The transformation of character which is the goal of all religious or mystical experience. It is the old theological term which denotes the integration or unification of the personality which merely begins with the acceptance of the Christian ideal and the identification with the Christian fellowship.

INSPIRATION. According to the common Christian doctrines the great prophets were " inspired " and the Bible was " given by inspiration." This, being interpreted, means that the prophets and writers of the Scriptures were regarded as passive instruments in the hands of God, who put his word into their mouths and dictated what they wrote. Our inquiry has shown that the experience of feeling oneself a passive instrument in the hands of some superpersonal force is by no means an uncommon one. We have explained it as an idea or thought process which after a period of incubation darts suddenly into consciousness and is felt as something external to the self (p. 92). The same mechanism is evident also in the auditory hallucinations of mental patients. This does not mean that those who interpret life in religious terms have no right to believe in the divine origin of their sacred writings. It does mean that we get into all sorts of trouble if we attempt to ascribe authority to any product of the mind merely because of the way in which it comes.

POSSESSION. The ancient explanation of abnormal phenomena such as inspiration and insanity, the one being ascribed to the presence of good and the other to the presence of evil spirits. This explanation is still current among spiritists.

From the Field of the Psychiatrist

PSYCHIATRY. That branch of medicine which has to do with the disorders of the personality. It is only within recent years that it has been receiving much attention and the number of psychiatrists is still relatively small. Of the approximately two thousand psychiatrists in this country only a few will be found in private practice in towns of less than fifty thousand.

PSYCHOPATHOLOGY. The basic science upon which the practice of psychiatry is founded. It has to do with the task of discovering the causative factors and the meaning of the different forms of personality disorder.

PSYCHOTHERAPY. The attempt to heal or cure by means of personal conferences with the patient (pp. 240–41). As distinguished from psychiatry it is not limited to the more severe disorders, and where psychiatry includes all that has to do with the more serious disorders, psychotherapy is limited to the realm of psychic influence.

PSYCHOANALYSIS. A special school of psychotherapy which follows the doctrines and techniques of Sigmund Freud of Vienna. In this country membership in the psychoanalytic associations is limited to members of the medical profession who have taken a course of training which includes a personal analysis.

MENTAL HYGIENE. A term brought into general use through the work of Clifford Beers. The mental hygiene movement grew out of his experience as a patient in a mental hospital and represents the efforts of psychiatrists to apply the insights derived from their work with the mentally ill to the task of prevention.

CLINICAL. Literally "bedside," a medical term used today somewhat loosely to denote actual experience with the sick. "Clinical training" is thus to be contrasted with instruction by books and lectures.

RAPPORT. An interpersonal relationship which permits the interflow of experience. In psychotherapeutic work a relationship of trust on the part of the patient toward the physician and of intelligent interest on the part of the physician toward the patient is a prerequisite. The Freudian term for this is "transference." For a consideration of this relationship see footnote to p. 161; also pp. 240–41.

NORMAL. Denotes conformity to some accepted standard. How that standard is determined is a matter on which practice differs. Very commonly what is usual is taken as the norm. In this case the norms are determined by getting the average of a large number of cases. Wherever, however, there is an agreement in regard to some objective or standard which is to be striven for, that objective is likely to be taken as the norm (pp. 164–65).

PATHOLOGICAL. A term which is applied to any deviation from health or normality. In considering a diseased condition it is important to distinguish between the real evil, such as a hostile germ or a foreign body or an instinctual indulgence clung to long after it ought to have been outgrown, and on the other hand curative processes by which nature seeks to eliminate the evil or mend the wound. The term "acute mental illness," as used in this book, denotes an emotional disturbance which like fever or inflammation in the physical organism represents an attempt to get rid of the evil (pp. 42–43, 53–57).

IDEATION. A term used in this book to denote content of thought as contrasted with "process" or "mechanism." The great advances in psychopathology made through Adolf Meyer and Sigmund Freud have come with the attempt to discover what the patient is thinking about and the origin and significance of his ideas (pp. 30 ff., 101 ff., 193–94).

PHANTASY. Undirected thinking or "daydreaming." Bleuler has attempted to distinguish between such thinking and "logical thought." He gave to it the name "autistic thinking." McDougall challenges this distinction and holds that from the standpoint of process all creative thinking is of the same associative type and is determined by the interests. The important distinction lies in the realm of values. Revery is constructive and creative when it is related to the individual's real objectives; worthless or dangerous when detached from those objectives. It is thus not the mere fact that an individual engages in daydreaming which gives occasion for concern, but the type of wishes or interests which become dominant.

AUTO–EROTISM. A term applied to solitary indulgence of the sex drive. It is used interchangeably with the term " masturbation," but it has frequently more particular reference to the phantasy life. For a consideration of this problem see pp. 36–37, 275 ff.

REPRESSION. A psychoanalytic term now widely current and frequently confused in popular speech with self-control. It denotes properly the exclusion from consciousness and from motor expression of painful or dangerous material by preventing its ideational presentation. It thus deals with troublesome instinctual claims by disowning them and refusing to acknowledge them. The result is that the disowned tendencies get by in disguised form and are indulged in secretly. From the standpoint of our inquiry it is important to notice that the evil to which Freud is referring lies precisely in the failure of self-control and in the resort to self-deception. The instinctual claims are not brought into the open and dealt with in the light of the requirements of the organized social self. They remain thus unassimilated and after the manner of unassimilated food they give the sufferer no peace until in some way or other they are taken care of. According to our findings such " complexes," as the Freudians call them, are not to be thought of as in the " unconscious." They are rather clamoring for attention (pp. 151–52).

DISSOCIATION. A term applied by Freud to the splitting off from the organized, social self of the disowned or repressed tendencies. These may form something in the nature of an independent organization. Janet and Morton Prince in their work with hysterical psychoneurotics found cases in which there was an emergence of secondary personalities. Between these secondary personalities and the normal self there was a break in the memory chain. Dissociation of this type is seldom encountered in the mental hospital. Bleuler, in coining the term " schizophrenia " (split mind), assumed that there was a splitting between idea and effect which was characteristic of the " dementia praecox " types. This is a doubtful point.

REGRESSION. A term used to denote the return to earlier levels of development which according to the view first advanced by Freud characterizes the dementia praecox types. Such a return he explained in terms of a " fixation " or blocking in the early years (cf. pp. 102 ff.). Jung introduced the idea of regression to a " racial unconscious " and emphasizes the constructive aspects of such experiences (pp. 106–7). Others use the term to denote merely the lapse into an inferior or primitive mode of behavior or ideation. This inquiry indicates that there can be such a thing as a journey to the lower regions which does not involve a moral letdown and that it may in fact represent an attempt at reorganization.

DISINTEGRATION. A term used to denote the fragmentation and demoralization which characterize such states as hebephrenic dementia praecox and distinguish them from the more hopeful catatonic types. Such fragmentation is generally reflected in disjointed thinking and loss of self-respect (pp. 37–43, 157).

HALLUCINATION. Commonly defined as a " mental impression of sensory vividness occurring without external stimulus." The commonest type is the " voices " so frequently encountered among mental patients. It is important to recognize that those who " hear voices " will usually dis-tinguish sharply between what they hear with their ears and what they hear " with their minds." They may describe the experience by saying that " it came to them," that " their conscience told them," or that they " had the impulse." Such " voices " we have regarded as merely an exaggerated form of the idea or thought process which after a period of incubation darts into consciousness and seems to come from an outside source. All normal persons have such experiences. To our patients such phenomena seem to be manifestations of the superpersonal and hence authoritative, or terrifying.

Hallucinations of vision, touch, taste and smell are also not uncommon, especially in the profounder disturbances. They may be understood by remembering that such a patient is living in a dream world where ideas have for him the value of reality. He is aware of and paying attention to processes which in the normal state are below the threshold of consciousness.

The fact that a person hears voices indicates that the deeper levels of the mental life are stirred. This in itself is neither good nor bad. Paul of Tarsus heard a voice on the road to Damascus and that fact is hardly to be regretted.

DELUSION. Is often defined as a " false belief." It is better to think of it as a belief, held to with emotional intensity by some individual, which is not shared by his fellows and serves to isolate him from them. Usually what is called " delusion " pertains to the individual's conception of himself and of his relationship to the external world. A hospital staff seldom calls a man deluded so long as his ideas, no matter how unusual, are shared by his group. Most of us today believe many things which are false and our beliefs, like a patient's delusions, may be determined by the requirements of the life-situation. They are part of the system of meanings, of the organization of attitudes and interpretations which enables us to reason and function (pp. 29, 43, 151–52).

ILLUSION. An erroneous interpretation which may be shared by the group. It is a false belief, but it does not isolate those who hold it. A mirage is an illusion. So also is the idea that the European nations, even if they were willing, would be able to pay off the war debts in gold.

REALITY. A term used to denote that which is essential, abiding, of central importance, capable of standing the test of experience. Reality is also defined as that which corrects our illusions. Beliefs regarding reality are the subject matter of metaphysics. The term " reality " is today much used in psychiatry. The Freudians speak of the " reality principle " as contrasted with the " pleasure principle." Some psychiatrists speak of the manic reaction as " flight into reality." As used by psychiatrists it means generally that which corrects illusions, and it is apt to be identified with that which one can see and feel. This inquiry has led us to the view that the catatonic who has become absorbed in a desperate inner struggle with what for him are the issues of life may be truly facing reality, and that reality is to be sought in the stuff that ideas are made of.

MENTAL AGE. The level of intelligence as determined by answers to questions of varying difficulty. These questions are standardized by means of answers obtained from many thousand children of different ages from three to 18 or 20 years. They were devised in the first place for use with the mentally deficient. By comparing his answers with the norms thus obtained a man may be said to have a mental age of ten years or of 14 years. Many such scales have been devised. The one most commonly used is the Stanford revision of the Binet-Simon test.

INTELLIGENCE QUOTIENT. The figure obtained by dividing the mental age rating of the person examined by the norm for his particular chronological age. Some difference of opinion exists as to what to use as the " basal year," or norm, for adults — whose intelligence quotient is not supposed to increase after the sixteenth year. According to the original standardization of the Stanford-Binet scale, based upon the answers given by several thousand California school children, 16 was the norm for the average adult. Subsequently, when this test was given to many thousands of men in connection with the Army entrance examinations, it was found that the average rating was somewhat less than 14 years. Immediately the cry went up that we were a nation of morons. Many careful psychologists have however drawn the more legitimate conclusion that the original norm was too high and are using 14 as the basal year (cf. F. L. Wells, *Mental Tests in Clinical Practice*, pp. 57–58).

DELINQUENCY. Misconduct in the case of individuals under 21 years of age which has brought them into conflict with the law. The term " criminal " is applied to the mature lawbreaker. As used in this book these terms are not applied to those who mean well and whose misconduct is due to intrapsychic conflict, but only to those whose will is antisocial (p. 143). The criminal and the delinquent come within the province of the courts, the educators and the psychiatrists.

MENTAL DEFICIENCY. Lack of native intelligence. The mentally deficient, or " feeble-minded," fall into three groups: the *idiots,* in whom intelligence is almost lacking, the *imbeciles* and the *morons*. It was at first customary to regard anyone with an intelligence quotient of less than 70, on the 16 year basis, as belonging in the feeble-minded group. Careful workers today are however accepting these ratings with much reserve.

The problem of mental deficiency is, of course, quite distinct from that of mental disorder and the feeble-minded are generally cared for in separate institutions. For the most part, however, these institutions are under the care of psychiatrists and in the census reports the feeble-minded are classified with the insane. The total number in institutions is probably less than 100,000.

MENTAL DISORDER. A term applied to peculiarities of belief and conduct which have set an individual apart from his fellows so that they look upon him as different and queer or find it impossible to live with him. The delinquents, in so far as they are not psychopathic, are gregarious, while the feeble-minded are generally amiable and happy. The mentally disordered fall into two major groups, those whose social maladjustments have a basis in demonstrable organic disease and those whose difficulties can be explained best in terms of unsolved personal problems.

Types of Mental Disorder

ORGANIC. Approximately one-third of the new patients brought each year to our mental hospitals have some disease of the brain which has so affected their social adjustments that they are said to have a " psychosis." Of this group the more important types are *general paresis,* which is a terminal stage of syphilis, and the structural changes, such as hardening of the arteries (*cerebral arterio-sclerosis*), which are responsible for the forgetfulness and other peculiarities of old people. These two groups together account for perhaps 22 per cent of the new admissions. Alcoholic poisoning accounts for most of the rest.

FUNCTIONAL. About two-thirds of the new admissions to mental hospitals are without demonstrable disease of brain or nervous tissue. The peculiarities of belief and conduct which have led to their commitment are explainable rather in terms of psychic disorganization. For a brief statement regarding the nature and causation of the functional disorders as revealed through this inquiry see pp. 151–58. Among these we may recognize the following types:

PSYCHOPATHIC PERSONALITY. A general term used somewhat loosely to denote poorly organized persons who have not gone so far as to have a " nervous breakdown." Here belong the irresponsible, the vacillating, the irritable, the perverted, etc.

PSYCHONEUROSIS. A term applied to severe intrapsychic conflict which manifests itself in certain definite symptoms but does not so far incapacitate the patient that he is unable to remain in touch with his group and sensitive to their opinions. Among the sub-types are *states of " irritable weakness "* (neurasthenia), *anxiety states, hysteria,* and *obsession-compulsion neuroses.* Of these four types the anxiety neuroses are to be regarded as transitional and the other three as attempts at equilibrium by means of certain compromise patterns. Due to the fact that my work in a mental hospital has not brought me into contact with many of these they are not dealt with in this book. The physician in private practice and the clergyman will, however, have many dealings with them.

EPILEPSY. A term applied to episodic disturbances of consciousness of a convulsive nature. The explanation of epilepsy is still a matter of controversy. No physical basis has as yet been demonstrated for true epilepsy. Epileptics are usually cared for in separate institutions. They have not been dealt with in this inquiry.

PSYCHOSIS. A term applied to those severer disturbances of the personality in which the patient is acting on premises and responding to symbols which his fellows do not recognize or accept. Among the psychoses three major groups may be mentioned. It is however to be noted that the prevailing classification has been made on a descriptive basis and not on the basis of the significant dynamic factors. It is therefore subject to much confusion as one goes from one group of diagnosticians to another. The descriptive groupings are not without significance but we would probably be better off if our psychiatric staffs would stop giving so much attention to a meaningless classification and more attention to the attempt to understand the real meaning of the experiences with which they are dealing. The following interpretations of the existing labels have been somewhat colored by our findings:

1. DEMENTIA PRAECOX. A label affixed to about 25 per cent of the new admissions and to about 50 per cent of the permanent population of our mental hospitals. It is an old Kraepelinian term and carries with it generally the implication of a bad prognosis. The term " schizophrenia," which is frequently used instead, was intended to place the emphasis upon the type of experience without reference to the prognosis. The common characteristic of this group is withdrawal from the external world and absorption in what is going on within. Our findings have indicated that it is important to distinguish dementia praecox as a *way of life* from dementia praecox as an *attempt at reorganization.* The following are the commonly recognized sub-types:

The *simple* type may be interpreted as denoting a way of life. It is represented in the individual who drifts off into a world of phantasy and easy pleasure-taking without putting up any determined resistance (pp. 28, 40, 157).

The *paranoic* type likewise denotes a way of life. It is represented in those who are unable to admit defeat or error and who distort their beliefs in order to save the conception of themselves and of their relationship to the external world on which their psychic structure is built. Such delusional formations tend to secure stabilization on an unsatisfactory basis. Among the paranoics we find two major types: those who resort to the device of blaming others for their difficulties and whose attitude is that of bitterness and hatred, and those who take refuge in a fictitious self-importance (pp. 29, 40–43, 154–56).

The *catatonic* type represents a desperate attempt at reorganization, following upon an awareness of danger, which tends either to make or break. We have seen that it bears a close relationship to the religious conversion experience (pp. 29, 40–43, 53–56, 79–82). Disturbances of this type may take the form of *stupor* or of *excitement*. They may also be looked upon as severer forms of the anxiety neurosis. For the types of solution which may follow a catatonic disturbance see pp. 159–62.

The *hebephrenic* type according to our findings represents the terminal stage of the drifting reaction or the demoralization which may follow upon an unsuccessful attempt at reorganization. It is the type in which the disowned tendencies get the upper hand and the unhappy individual becomes more and more disintegrated. His speech is apt to be lacking in logical sequence and he tends to become silly and uninhibited and indecent and to have bizarre ideas (pp. 37–38, 40–43).

2. MANIC–DEPRESSIVE. A label affixed to about ten per cent of our new admissions. Kraepelin, who coined this term, held that this disorder was characterized by mood swings either in the direction of exaltation or of depression, with a tendency to swing from one extreme to the other. He therefore spoke of the " manic phase " and of the " depressed phase " of the manic-depressive psychosis. The Freudians explain it as a reaction in which the harsh " super ego " (conscience) and the repressed tendencies become detached from each other and express themselves in alternating periods. This inquiry indicates that cases in which there is a swing from one extreme to the other are the exception rather than the rule and that the two phases constitute totally different reaction patterns. Even though these may sometimes occur within the same individual, it would seem best to keep them separate.

The *manic* reaction is one of active concern about the external world. A patient of this type is self-confident, overactive, euphoric, self-important and self-assertive. Where the schizophrenic is living in a world of phantasy, the manic is living out his daydreams. Where the schizophrenic is concerned with *ideas* which seem to come from a superpersonal source, the manic feels himself *doing* things he can't account for except on the basis of superhuman strength. In some cases the manic reaction follows upon unexpected success in the case of an individual who feels inwardly insecure. It is to be noted that excited catatonics frequently have manic characteristics and that cases which in one hospital are labeled " manic " will in another institution be classified as " dementia praecox, catatonic type." Manic reactions are often spoken of as " flight into reality." It seems better to regard them as escape into self-assertive activity. While such reactions tend to wear off and the patient comes out in relatively good condition, they tend to recur. In many cases this reaction represents the breaking through of repressed tendencies with a resulting disorganization which expresses itself in disjointed, flighty speech.

The *depression* reaction differs from the stuporous catatonic only in the depth of the regression and in the presence or absence of the more malignant features. The reaction pattern is that of self-blame and despair. It is an extreme form of the blues.

3. INVOLUTIONAL MELANCHOLIA. A term applied to depressions and to agitated states which occur in the fifth or sixth decades of life. It is commonly assumed that such troubles are connected with the physiological changes incidental to the menopause in women and the corresponding period in men. It seems rather more probable that they are due to difficulty in making the grade in the new level of development which needs to be attained at this period. From the standpoint of reaction patterns there seems no reason to retain this grouping.

INDEX

Affect, 29ff., 56, 60, 68, 79ff., 151
definition of, 305
Alexander, Franz, 106, 143, 202–3
Assimilation of new experience, 149, 151–52
Atonement, doctrine of the, 204–6
Attention, narrowing of, 79, 117, 121
Attitude, 56, 69, 81, 106, 151–52, 171–72, 194, 269, 277, 279, 284
definition of, 305
Auto-erotism, 25–26, 36–38, 272–80, 283
definition of, 311
Auto-hypnosis, 79, 117
Automatism, 92

Belief, 29, 80–81, 138–39, 151–52, 156–58, 170–74, 228, 230–33
Birth control, 274–75
Body and mind, 21–27, 194–95
Bundy, Walter E., 130, 136
Bunyan, John, 69–71, 94–95

Cabot, Richard C., 8, 251–52
Cadbury, H. J., 133
Campbell, C. M., 8, 29, 240–41
Case, S. J., 129, 131
Catatonia: see Dementia praecox
Chaplaincies in mental hospitals, 6, 8–9, 222, 251–63
Character, 142–62, 164
definition of, 303
Christianity, challenge to liberal, 235–37
Church
current trends in liberal, 232–35
function of, 213–15, 224–26, 232
Clinical
definition of, 310
training for theological students, 10, 251–63

Coe, George A., 92–94, 117
Collective
ideology, 108–9
unconscious, 106–7
Complex, 149, 152
Compromise devices, 154, 174, 202–7
Concealment reactions, 29, 35–36, 40, 43, 152, 154–58, 173–74, 202–7, 228, 268–69
Conflict, intra-psychic
acute, may be essential to growth, 53–57, 59–82, 89–91, 112, 121, 202–6, 266
as explanation of functional mental disorder, 5, 24–27, 102–6, 111, 113, 121, 144
determined by social requirements, 102–5, 108–9, 151–52, 170–76, 178–80, 209–10, 275–77
forces involved in, 27, 90–91, 106–7, 108–9, 137–38, 149–50, 175, 178–79, 209
pathological only when attended by sense of isolation, 268
types of solution, 5, 28–29, 43, 153–62, 201–2, 207, 211, 227–28, 244, 268, 280–81
Conscience, 35, 105–6, 143–44, 151–52, 171–76
definition of, 306
Consciousness, 102 ff., 151–52, 158–59, 161, 175, 189
definition of, 303–4
Conversion experience
as solution of intra-psychic conflict, 75–79, 89–93, 199, 280–81
definition of, 308
disappearance of, from present-day liberal churches, 234

317

relationship to acute type of mental disorder, 5, 59–61, 79–82, 121, 158–59, 202–6
types of, 207–8
value of, 85, 92–93, 95, 199, 205–6, 291–93
Cooley, Charles H., 171
Cosmic catastrophe, ideas of
characteristic of acute mental disorder, 3, 32–34, 39, 55, 168–70
explanation of, 103–4, 117, 197–98
found in certain men of religious genius, 62, 71, 72–75, 127–41
Cosmic identification
associated with ideas of cosmic catastrophe, 3, 32–34, 39, 55, 168–70
explanation of, 117, 120–21, 138–40, 197–98
Cotton, H. A., 100–1
Criminal
law, 205
types, 143
Cross, doctrine of, 204–6
Culture, 186, 192, 214, 252
definition of, 306

Dante Alighieri, 15
Death, ideas of, 34, 39, 75, 117–20, 132–34, 296
Delacroix, Henri, 95–96, 118
Delinquency, 153, 282–83
definition of, 313
Delinquents
characteristics of, 163ff., 173
contrasted with the psychopathic, 28, 143–46, 173–74
treatment of, 270
types of, 143
Delusion, 29, 35–36, 40–43, 101–2, 104, 152, 155–57
definition of, 312
Dementia praecox, 4, 15–57, 104, 110–11, 157–60
definition of, 315–16
catatonic type, 4, 40–48, 110–11, 158–60
definition of, 316
hebephrenic type, 37, 40–43, 110–11, 157–60
definition of, 316
paranoic type, 29, 35–36, 40–43, 104, 155–57

definition of, 316
simple type, 28, 40, 43, 157–58
definition of, 315
Depravity, total, 193
Depression, 34, 109–10, 158–59
see also Manic-depressive
Desire, 102–9, 149–50, 190–91, 202–3
definition of, 304–5
Determinism, 185
Development, types of, 158–59
Dewey, John, 171, 182, 304
Dicks, R. L., 252
Disintegration, 37, 40–43, 104, 110–11, 157–58
definition of, 312
Disinterestedness, scientific, 187
Dollard, John, 186

Economic misfortune and mental health, 271
Emotion, 31ff., 56, 63, 74–75, 77, 79, 143, 194, 208, 226
definition of, 305
Empiricism
as an approach to ethics, 166ff.
in scientific procedure, 184–85
Environment as a factor in mental illness, 22
Epilepsy, 90
definition of, 315
Erotic involvement in schizophrenia, 36–37
Eruptive reactions, 43, 54–56, 79–82, 90–91, 110–11, 158–59, 204, 207–8
Escape devices, 173–74
see also Concealment
Estrangement, sense of: see Isolation
Ethical values as functions of social relationships, 179–80
Evangelistic task of church, 272–73, 281–82
Expiation, 202–6
Ezekiel, 72

Family as unit in church organization, 225, 284
see also Parents
Fear, 3, 29, 32–34, 60, 80, 109–10, 144, 152, 158–59, 167, 169, 205, 212, 268, 273, 279, 300
Feeling, 48ff., 56, 63–64, 66ff., 69, 73, 79–80, 91, 92, 95, 176, 190, 192, 194, 196, 267–68